INTERMITTENT FASTING FOR WOMEN AND AUTOPHAGY

The Smartest Guide to Lose Weight by Eating Healthy and For Heal Your Body Through the Self-Cleansing Process of Autophagy

Respective authors own all copyrights not held by the publisher.

The information herein is offered for informational purposes solely and is universal as so. The presentation of the information is without a contract or any type of guarantee assurance.

The trademarks that are used are without any consent, and the publication of the trademark is without permission or backing by the trademark owner. All trademarks and brands within this book are for clarifying purposes only and are owned by the owners themselves, not affiliated with this document.

Table of Contents

INTRODUCTION

Intermittent Fasting (IF) refers to dietary ingestion patterns that entail not eating or severely limiting calories for a delayed interval. There are a variety of subgroups of discontinuous fasting. These include having singular dietary variety every day, a long time, or daily. This has come to be a very prominent subject in the science community due to the possible benefits on health which are constantly being discovered.

WHAT IS INTERMITTENT FASTING (IF)?

Fasting or instances of deliberate restraint from nutrition have been rehearsed throughout the world for quite a very long time. Discontinuous fasting with the target of enhancing wellbeing is refreshing. Discontinuous fasting involves limiting the entry of nourishment during a specified timeframe and can exclude some progressions into the true food resources you're eating. As of this moment, the most frequently recognized IF conventions are a daily 16 hour fast, then fasting for a whole day, once or twice a week. Irregular fasting can be regarded as an eating style where people follow our Palaeolithic tracker/gatherer predecessors. The current model of a structured application of intermittent fasting might improve many health concerns, from life length and aging. Regardless if IF breaks traditional lifestyle and routine program, the science is encouraging less eating and more time fasting. Otherwise, it just compares to the normal breakfast, lunch, and dinner model. Listed below are just two fantasies that are relevant to intermittent fasting.

Fantasy 1 - You must eat 3 meals per day. This "principle" is routine in Western civilization and wasn't created or determined by evidence for enhanced health. However, it was a simple example made by pilgrims, which eventually became the norm. Not only is there a lack of a logical system of justification from the three meal a day version, but ongoing examinations also fasting to be excellent for human health. One study suggested that one meal each day using an identical measure of daily calories is better for weight loss reduction and body synthesis than 3 meals daily. This finding was the vital thought that was extrapolated into intermittent fasting. However, most people deciding to begin IF may believe it's best to eat 1-2 meals a day.

Legend 2 - You need breakfast; it is the most important meal of this day. Several bogus cases about the requirement for breakfast have been perpetuated. The most frequently recognized instances are "breakfast aids your digestion" and "breakfast increases nourishment ingestion later in the day". These instances have been discredited with results suggesting that skipping breakfast did not reduce digestion and it did not build nourishment intake at lunch and dinner. It's better to perform intermittent fasting while having breakfast;

nevertheless, some men and women believe it's easier to get a late breakfast or bypass it large.

The simple program and promising effects of time-confined encouraging may allow it to be an unbelievable alternative for weight loss and ceaseless illness counteractive action across the board. While executing this seminar, it may be great in the first place to have a lesser fasting-to-eating ratio like 12/12 hours and in the very long term stir your way around 16/8 hours.
The fundamental question about intermittent fasting:

Is there some nourishment or refreshment I'm permitted to expend while still on intermittent fasting? Except if you're performing the altered fasting 5:2 eating regimen (referenced above), then do your best not to consume or ingest anything that contains calories. Water, black espresso, and some other nourishments/drinks which don't include carbs are ok to consume through a fasting period. Truth be told, adequate water entrance is essential throughout IF and a few say that ingesting dark espresso whilst fasting empowers diminishing appetite.

Irregular Fasting is now a well-known approach to shed weight quickly. Whatever the case, a lot of people will need to understand how discontinuous fasting operate and just how precisely it does function. At the stage when you go to get an off-beat timeframe without eating, your body alters the way it produces compounds and hormones, which can be great for fat disputes. These are the main fasting benefits and the way they achieve those benefits.

Hormones construct the assumption of metabolic capabilities including the pace at which you have fat. The development hormone is made by your own body and progresses the breakdown of fat from the body to provide energy. At the stage when you fast for some time, your body starts to expand its growth hormone production. Likewise, fasting tries to reduce the amount of insulin within the circulatory system, assuring your body absorbs fat rather than putting it away.

A momentary fast that keeps moving 12-72 hours increases the digestion and adrenaline levels, which makes you increase the number of calories consumed daily. Moreover, those who fast likewise achieve more outstanding vitality through enlarged adrenaline, forcing them not to feel tired in spite of the fact they are not getting calories and. Regardless of how you might feel like, fasting ought to bring about diminished energy, the body makes up for this, assuring a fatty consuming method.

A great many men and women who consume every 3-5 hours, basically eat sugar instead of fat. Fasting for longer intervals makes your digestion to swallow fat. Ahead of the conclusion of a 24-hour fast day, your body has spent glycogen stores in the very first few hours and has spent approximately 18 of the hour's intensive fat stores in the body. For any person who's routinely lively, yet at precisely the exact same time struggles with fat misfortune, discontinuous fasting may construct fat misfortune without inclining an exercise program, or correct an eating regime program.

Another benefit of discontinuous fasting is that it resets the body. A day or so without ingesting affects an individual's cravings, which makes them feel excited after a time. On the off chance you struggle with consistently needing nutrition, intermittent fasting may empower your body to adapt to occasions of not eating and help you not to feel hungry constantly. Quite a few people see that they begin to consume more valuable and progressively controlled eating regimens, whenever they fast irregularly 1 day every seven days.

Discontinuous fasting changes, are suggested for approximately one day consistently. On this day, a person might have a fluid supplement packed smoothie or a low-calorie alternative. Since the body changes using an intermittent fasting strategy, this normally is not important. Discontinuous fasting reduces fat chops normally from the body, by simply altering the digestion to different fat rather than muscle or sugar. It's been viably used by many people and it's an easy technique to rolling out an improvement that is beneficial. For any person who struggles with stubborn fat and can be worn out on habitual abstaining from excessive food intake, intermittent fasting provides a very simple and productive option for fat misfortune and a more advantageous method of life.

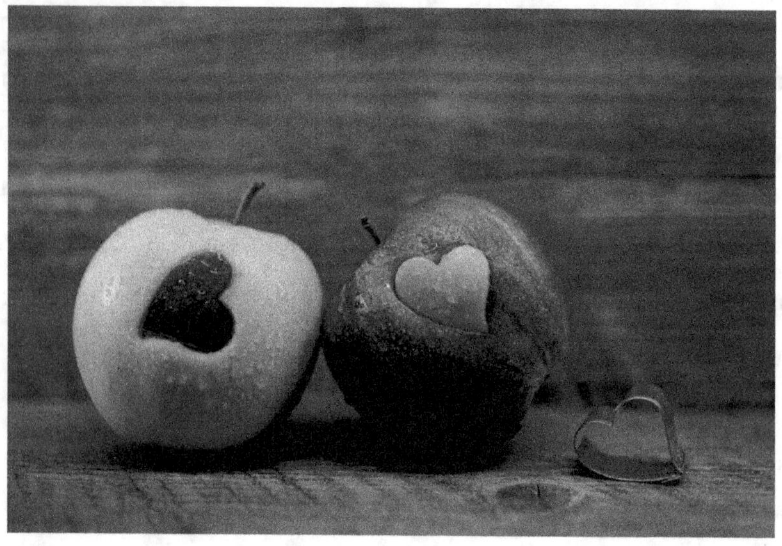

CHAPTER 1
What's INTERMITTENT FASTING?

Fasting is another thought. For a long time, people have temporarily limited their nutrition intake for rigorous explanations. In the past few decades, discontinuous fasting -- for those who do not consume for somewhere in the assortment of 16 -- 48 hours (or longer) -- has been a matter of interest because of its mind-boggling effects on illness and aging.

Irregular Fasting (IF) is now among the world's most notable wellness and health routines.

Folks are using it more to enhance their health and disentangle their manners of life.

Numerous studies indicate it may influence your entire body and cerebrum and might even help you live longer.

This is a definitive student's guide for intermittent fasting.

What's discontinuous fasting?

Irregular fasting is the method of biking all through instances of eating and eating. Although people do experience weight loss with discontinuous fasting, it's to a lesser extent a regular eating arrangement and to a larger degree a way for living to obtain some mind-blowing health rewards.

Discontinuous fasting (IF) is an eating plan that spans between instances of eating and fasting.

It does not signify which nourishments you need to consume; however, rather, it's when you need to consume them.

In this respect, it's anything but an eating regime from the normal sense, yet more exactly portrayed as an eating style.

Fundamental intermittent fasting plans incorporate daily 16-hour fasts or fasting for 24 hours, twice each week.

Fasting has been coaching all through human improvement. Old tracker gatherers did not have grocery shops, iceboxes or nutrition available annually. Occasionally, they could not find anything to eat.

Subsequently, people designed to have the choice to work without nutrition for enlarged timeframes.

Truth be told, fasting every now and then, is much more ordinary than always ingesting 3--4 (or even more) meals daily.

Fasting is likewise routinely accomplished for rigorous or religious motives, integrating into Islam, Christianity, Judaism, and Buddhism.

Rundown irregular fasting (IF) is an eating plan that spans between instances of eating and fasting. It is currently well known in the health network.

Discontinuous fasting methods.

There are a couple of different procedures for performing discontinuous fasting -- most of which include things like parting daily or weekly to fasting and eating intervals.

The fasting period frames: you consume next to nothing or with no stretch of the imagination.

All these would be very well-known approaches:

• The 16/8 plan: Also known as the lean gains tradition; it involves skipping breakfast and restricting your daily eating interval to 8 hours; by way of instance, 1--9 p.m. Now you fast for 16 hours at the center.

• Eat-stop-Eat: Including fasting for 24 hours, even more than once each week, for example by not needing dinner daily before dinner the next day.

• The 5:2 eating regularly: With these strategies, you consume only 500--600 calories on two non-sequential times of this week; nevertheless, eat the other five days.

By lessening your calorie intake, these techniques must lead to weight loss if you do not repay by ingesting considerably more during the ingestion time frames.

Numerous individuals find the 16/8 approach as the least complicated; typically maintainable and simplest to stick to. It is also very mainstream.

Outline there, are a couple of unique approaches to performing discontinuous fasting. Each of them divides the week or week into fasting and eating intervals.
How does it affect your cells and hormones?

At the stage when you fast, a few things happen in your own body on the mobile and nuclear levels.

For example, your body changes hormone levels to create burn muscle versus fat progressively offered.

Your cells also start significant repair procedures and adjust the outflow of attributes.

Here are a couple of changes that occur in your body if you fast:

• Human Growth Hormone (HGH): The levels of growth hormone soar, expanding up to 5-overlay. This has advantages for fat loss misfortune and muscle gain, to provide a few examples.

• Insulin: Insulin affectability is enhanced and amounts of insulin fall radically. Reduced insulin levels make muscle to fat ratio progressively reduced.

• Cellular fix: Once fasted, your cells begin cell repair forms. This comprises of autophagy, where cells procedure expels useless and old proteins which advances inside cells.

• Gene articulation: You can find changes at the capacity of attributes diagnosed, with lifetime and confidence from illness.

All these alterations in hormone levels, mobile capacity, and excellent articulation are liable for the health care benefits of intermittent fasting.

Outline: When you fast, human growth hormone levels go up and insulin levels return. Your body's cells also alter the announcement of attributes and begin considerable cell repair forms.

An extremely successful weight loss tool

Weight reduction is the most frequently recognized explanation behind people trying intermittent fasting. By causing you to eat fewer suppers, intermittent fasting may prompt a programmed reduction in calorie entrance.

Furthermore, discontinuous fasting affects hormone levels to promote weight loss.

Notwithstanding bringing insulin down and enlarging growth hormone levels, it assembles the coming of the fat intensive hormone norepinephrine (noradrenaline).

On account of those alterations in hormones, transient fasting can enlarge your metabolic rate by 3.6--14 percent.

By assisting you to eat less and eat more calories, intermittent fasting induces weight reduction by altering the 2 sides of their calorie condition.

Studies show that discontinuous fasting may be an incredibly miraculous weight reduction device.

A 2014 research study found this ingestion example may result in 3--8 percent weight loss over 3--24 weeks, and it is a remarkable amount, compared with most weight-loss beliefs.

In a similar report, people also lost 4--7 percent of the midriff perimeter, demonstrating a remarkable loss of dangerous gut fat which develops around your organs and triggers the disease.

Another research suggested that discontinuous fasting induces less muscle misfortune compared to the standard methods of persistent calorie confinement.

In any case, do not forget that the principal reason for its abundance is that intermittent fasting induces you to consume fewer calories and large. In case you gorge and consume substantial sums throughout your eating intervals, you might not lose any weight at all.

Rundown intermittent fasting can marginally encourage digestion while assisting you to consume fewer calories. It is an exceptionally strong approach to lose weight and belly fat.

There are diverse intermittent fasting methods. All these are:

• 5:2: This approach allows you to consume typically five times each week. The other two days will be the fasting times, although you do even now eat. Just keep it somewhere in the assortment of 500 and 600 calories.

• Eat-stop-eat: With this, you limit all nutrition for 24 hours, even more than once each week.

• 16/8: You consume the entirety of your own daily calories within an abbreviated period -- normally 6 to 8 hours and fast for your remaining 14 to 16 hours. You can do this frequently, or a few times per week.

• Bulletproof irregular fasting most carefully takes following the 16/8 plan, yet with a single essential comparison: you drink a few bulletproof coffees at the very first portion of the day. It is a wise hack to maintain the cravings for food while staying in the fasting condition. Whatever the case, more about this later.

Medical benefits of discontinuous fasting

At this stage, if you don't consume any nourishment to get a set timeframe daily, you do your own body and your brain a great mess. It does well from a developmental angle. For most time in history, folks were not ingesting three nourishing dinners every day, along with brushing on bites. Instead, folks developed in situations where there was not a great deal of nourishment, and they figured out the way to thrive when fasting. Nowadays, we do not have to pursue nutrition (even though pursuing your own meat is anything but an ill-conceived idea!). Or perhaps we undergo a sizable part of our times prior to PCs, and we consume at whatever stage we desire -- although our bodies are not adjusted to this behavior.

Shifting into a discontinuous fasting diet develops the points of confinement and lifts your display in a variety of ways. Listed below are a part of the extraordinary benefits of intermittent fasting:

• Encourages weight loss

• Increases vitality

• Promotes cell repair and autophagy (if your own body expends faulty tissue in order to make new components)

• reduces insulin resistance and guarantees against type 2 diabetes

• Lowers terrible cholesterol

• interrupts life length

- shield against neurodegenerative maladies, by way of instance, Alzheimer's and Parkinson's

• Improves lifts and memory mind work

• Makes cells more powerful

Numerous studies are performed on intermittent fasting, with 2 animals and people.

All these examinations have shown that it may have revolutionary advantages for weight reduction and the health of body and mind. It may even help you with living longer.

Here are the key medical benefits of discontinuous fasting:

• Weight hazards: As referenced previously, discontinuous fasting can help you with becoming healthier and paunch fat, without needing to intentionally limit calories (1, 13Trusted Source).

• Insulin barrier: irregular fasting may diminish insulin resistance, bringing down sugar --6 percent and fasting insulin levels by 20--31 percent, which should guarantee against type 2 diabetes.

• Inflammation: Several assessments show decreases in markers of aggravation, an integral driver of many incessant infections.

• Heart health: Intermittent fasting may reduce "awful" LDL cholesterol, blood glucose, incendiary markers, sugar, and insulin obstruction -- most of the risk factors for coronary disease.

• Cancer: Animal analyses suggest that intermittent fasting can expend malignant growth.

• Brain health: Intermittent fasting Increases the cerebrum hormone BDNF and might assist the growth of new cells. It may likewise guarantee against Alzheimer's illness.

• Anti-maturing: Irregular fasting can extend life expectancy. Studies have shown that fasted rodents dwelt 36--83% more.

Recall that mining is still in its start phases. A significant number of those investigations were small, current moment or conducted in animals. Quite a few inquiries currently can not appear to get answered in more outstanding human tests.

Rundown intermittent fasting may have numerous benefits for your entire body and cerebrum. It can induce weight reduction and might reduce your threat of type 2 diabetes, coronary disease, and disorder. It may likewise help make your healthy lifestyle simpler.

Eating nicely is simple, yet it might very well be incredibly tough to maintain.

One of the principal impediments is all the work necessary to prepare for and cook strong suppers.

Irregular fasting can make matters easier since you do not need to strategies; just concoct or keep following the exact same amount of dinners as previously.

Hence, discontinuous fasting is known among the life-hacking swarm, as it enhances your health while at precisely the exact same time, streamlining your daily life concurrently.

A summary of the substantial benefits of discontinuous fasting is that it makes intelligent dieting simpler. You will find fewer dinners that you need to plan, cook, and watch after.

Who must perform or avoid it?

Irregular fasting is not for everyone.

If you are underweight or possess a background marked with dietary difficulties, you shouldn't fast without counseling with health proficient first.

These scenarios might be very well harmful and out.

If girls quickly?

There is some evidence that intermittent fasting might not be as beneficial for women, all things considered, as it is for guys.

For example, one study demonstrated its enhanced insulin efficiency in men but declined sugar control in women.

Even though human analyses at this stage are inaccessible, observations in rodents have found that intermittent fasting may cause female rodents anorexic, masculinized, barren and lead them to miss cycles.

There are various story reports of women whose menstrual period stopped when they started doing IF and returned into normal if they continued their previous eating style.

Thus, women should be more careful with intermittent fasting.

They should pursue distinct rules, like slipping to the practice and stopping immediately on the off possibility if they have any problems such as amenorrhea (nonappearance of a female cycle).

With the off probability, you have problems with ripeness too, and as you are trying to envision, think about holding off irregular fasting for now. This eating style is probably likewise an ill-conceived notion in the event you're pregnant or breastfeeding.

Rundown individuals that are underweight or have a past full of dietary issues shouldn't fast. There's also some evidence that intermittent fasting may be dangerous to certain women.

Safety and Negative Effects

Yearning is the main response of discontinuous fasting.

You may likewise feel weak and your cerebrum might not implement as you are used to.

This may only be impermanent since it could put aside some attempt for the body to adapt to the new feast program.

The off probability, that you have an ailment, you need to seek advice from your primary care doctor before trying irregular fasting.

This is especially important in case you

• Have diabetes.

• suffer from sugar rule.

• Have a low heartbeat.

• are on medication.

• Are underweight.

• Have a past full of dietary issues.

• Are a woman Who's trying to imagine.

• Are a woman with a past full of amenorrhea.

• Are pregnant or breastfeeding.

Discontinuous fasting includes a remarkable health profile. There's nothing insecure about not eating for a while in the event you're strong and well-supported generally.

Synopsis: the most frequently recognized manifestation of discontinuous fasting is appetite. People with specific ailments shouldn't fast without counseling with a professional first.

Starting

Odds are that you have only done numerous intermittent fasts during your lifetime.

On the off probability that you have had dinner, or you slept later than you had before lunch the next day, or you have presumably as of today fasted for 16+ hours.

A couple of individuals intuitively consumes this way. They essentially do not feel hungry during the first portion of the day.

Numerous people consider the 16/8 plan the least challenging and most economical way of discontinuous fasting -- you need to try this practice first.

In the event that you believe its easy and feel good throughout the period, at this point, possibly give a transferring shot to additionally grown fasts like 24-hour fasts one-two times per week (Eat-Stop-Eat), or simply eating 500--600 calories 1--2 days out of every week (5:2 eating regular).

Another methodology is to simply quit at whatever stage it is advantageous -- basically skip suppers again when you are not eager or do not have the chance to cook.

There is no persuasive reason to pursue a coordinated intermittent fasting plan to recognize probably some of the benefits.

Examine the diagnosis together with the several methodologies and find something which you enjoy, and which accommodates your schedule.

Rundown is prescribed to start with this 16/8 plan, at this point; possibly later, proceed ahead to more fasts. It is crucial to try and finds a plan that is appropriate for you.

Can it be a fantastic idea for one to try this?

Discontinuous fasting is not something that anyone must do.

It is just among numerous means of life methods that could enhance your wellbeing. Eating real nutrition, practicing and coping with your remainder areas are the most important factors to focus on.

The off probability that you don't care for fasting; at that point, you can safely dismiss this guide and continue doing what works for you.

At the end of the day, there's no one-size-fits-all arrangement with respect to sustenance. The ideal diet for you is one you're able to adhere to over the long haul.

Discontinuous fasting is exceptional for certain people. The very best way to discover that bunch you own a location with, would be to give it a shot.

The occasion you are feeling good when fasting and watch it as a maintainable way of eating, it very well might be an integral advantage to get fit and improve your wellness.

Famous Tactics to Do Intermittent Fasting

Discontinuous fasting has been quite trendy as of late.

It is professed to induce weight loss, improve metabolic health and perhaps even expand life expectancy.

Anyone might anticipate given that the prominence, a couple of different sorts/techniques for intermittent fasting are contrived.

Each one of them may be strong, yet which one fits best depends upon the individual.

INTERMITTENT FASTING AND WOMEN

Perhaps not like a daily caloric reduction diet, but discontinuous fasting increases digestion. This is well established from an endurance perspective. On the off probability, we do not consume; the body put energy away as fuel together until we're able to stay living to detect another feast. Hormones permit the body to change vitality resources from nutrition to muscle.

Studies reveal this miracle clearly. For example, four days of nonstop fasting enlarged Basal metabolic rate by 12 percent. Amounts of this synapse norepinephrine, which divides the body for action, is enlarged by 117 percent. Unsaturated fats are enlarged by over 370 percent as the body shifts from absorbing nutrition to storing fat.

Unlike a continuous calorie-confinement diet, intermittent fasting does not consume muscles. In 2010, experts studied a group of subjects that underwent 70 days of daily fasting (ate a single afternoon and fasted the next). Many of them started at

52.0 kg and ended in 51.9 kg. Therefore, there was no reduction of muscles; nevertheless, they dropped 11.4 percent of fat and found substantial updates in LDL cholesterol and triglyceride levels.

Throughout fasting, the body typically generates progressively human growth hormone to safeguard slender bones and muscles. Bulk is often protected till muscle to fat ratio drops under 4 percent. This manner, the huge majority aren't at risk of muscle-squandering whilst performing discontinuous fasting.

Turns around insulin resistance, type two diabetes, and fatty liver.

Type 2 diabetes is a condition where there's essentially an inordinate quantity of sugar from the body, to the point that the mobiles can not react to insulin and consume any more sugar in the bloodstream (insulin obstruction), causing high glucose level. Furthermore, the liver becomes piled with fat since it tries to eliminate the prosperity sugar by altering it over to and putting it away.

Subsequently, to reverse this ailment, two things will need to happen:

• First, stop putting sugar into the entire body.

• Second, eat the rest of the sugar off.

The finest diet to do this is really a low-sugar, moderate-protein, also high-solid fat eating regime similarly called ketogenetic diet plan. (Remember that starch increases sugar the most, protein marginally, and fat at the least.) That's the reason why a low-carb diet can help decrease the burden of glucose. For certain people, this is enough to change insulin resistance and type two diabetes. Be as it may, in acute scenarios, diet alone is not adequate.

Shouldn't something be said about exercise? Exercise can help ignite the elimination of sugar in the skeletal tissues; nevertheless, not in all cells and organs like greasy liver. Evidently, the clinic is important, yet to extract the prosperity sugar in the organs, there's the requirement to "starve" cells.

Irregular fasting can attain this. That's the motive; people referred to fasting psychologists or even detox. It tends to be a wonderful asset to eliminate this substantial variety of overabundances. It's the fastest method to reduce blood sugar and insulin levels, and ultimately shifting insulin resistance, type two diabetes, and fatty liver.

Coincidentally, taking insulin for type 2 diabetes does not deal with the most important driver of the matter, which can be overabundance sugar within the body. The facts show that insulin will reduce the glucose in the bloodstream, bringing about reduced blood sugar; yet where can the sugar move to? The liver is going to change everything into fat in the liver and fat from the mid-region. Patients that go on insulin, often end up putting on more fat, which reduces their diabetes.

Upgrades heart health

As time goes on, higher blood sugar from type two diabetes may damage the nerves and veins which control the center. The longer one has diabetes, the higher the chances that coronary disease will come up. By bringing down sugar through discontinuous fasting, the threat of cardiovascular disease and stroke is similarly diminished.

Moreover, discontinuous fasting was observed to enhance cardiovascular problems, increase LDL (awful) cholesterol, blood glucose, and incendiary markers associated with numerous ceaseless ailments.

Lifts intellectual art

Numerous studies revealed fasting has many neurologic benefits including center and consideration, reaction time, instantaneous memory, discernment, and the era of new synapses. Mice ponders also indicated that discontinuous fasting reduces cerebrum annoyance and avoids the unwanted effects of Alzheimer's disease.

What is the benefit of occasional fasting?

Craving goes down

We normally feel cravings for food about four hours following dinner. On the off possibility we fast for 24 hours, does this suggest our craving senses will multiply and be increasingly severe? Obviously not.

Numerous people are concerned that fasting will result in an outrageous appetite and laughing. Studies have shown that on the following a long time after a one-day fast, there is certainly a 20% growth in the caloric entrance. Whatever the situation, together with continued fasting, yearning, and appetite surprisingly decrease.

Craving comes in waves. In case we do not do anything, the longing disperses invariably. Drinking tea (numerous sorts) or java (with or without caffeine) is frequently enough to fend it off.

Be as it may, it's best to drink it darkish nevertheless a teaspoon or two of cream or creamer will not activate a great deal of insulin response. Attempt not to use any sorts of sugars or counterfeit sugars. On the off chance that essential, bone soup may similarly be obtained through fasting.

Glucose does not crash

Now and then folks stress that sugar will drop tremendously low through fasting and they'll acquire unsteady and sweat-soaked. This does not really happen as sugar is strongly observed from the human body and there are assorted tools to keep it at the best possible variety. Through fasting, the body begins to separate glycogen from the liver to release sugar. This occurs each late night during our break.

In case that we fast for more than 24-36 hours, then glycogen stores become emptied and the liver is likely to create new glucose using glycerol that is due to the breakdown of fat (a process known as gluconeogenesis). Besides utilizing sugar, our synapses can similarly use ketones for energy. Ketones are generated when fat is utilized and they're able to provide around 75 percent of the cerebrum's energy requirements (another 25 percent from sugar).

The primary exemption is for the people that are taking diabetic insulin and meds. You must initially advise your primary care doctor as the dosages will probably be diminished as you're fasting. Another thing, on the off probability that you just overmedicate, and hypoglycemia occurs, you ought to have some sugar to flip around it. This may break the speed and ensure it is counterproductive.

The first light miracle

After a period of fasting, especially toward the start of the day, a couple of men and women experience elevated blood sugar. This afternoon break marvel is an aftereffect of this circadian rhythm whereby just before stimulating, the body exerts considerable levels of a few hormones to prepare for the up and coming day -

• Adrenaline - to provide the body with some power

• Growth hormone - to help mend and create fresh protein

• Glucagon - to transfer sugar from the liver into the blood to be used as energy

• Cortisol, the stress hormone - to initiate your system

All these hormones leading to the first portion of the daylight hours, in the point fall to bring down amounts over the course of the day. In non-diabetics, the degree of the sugar rise is small, and the huge majority will not see it. Be as it can, for most of the diabetics, there may be a visible spike in blood sugar since the liver dumps sugar to the blood.

This will happen in broadened fasts too. Whenever there isn't any nourishment, insulin levels stay low while the liver releases some of its fat and sugar. This is common rather than being a terrible thing by any means. The greatness of this spike will diminish since the liver proves to be enlarged with fat and sugar.

Who shouldn't do intermittent fasting?

• Girls who are pregnant, or will be pregnant, or are breastfeeding.

• People that are malnourished or underweight.

• Kids under 18 years of age and older folks.

• People who have gout.

• People who have gastroesophageal celiac disease (GERD).

• People who have dietary issues should initially seek advice from their primary care doctors.

• People that are taking diabetic meds and insulin should seek advice from their primary care doctors as dimensions ought to be diminished.

• People that are taking prescriptions should initially advise with their primary care doctors as the preparation of medication may be affected.

• People who are feeling pressured or possess cortisol problems shouldn't fast since fasting is just another stressor.

• People that are having exceptionally challenging duties most days of the week shouldn't fast.

How to Get Ready for Irregular Fasting?

The off chance that anyone is considering starting discontinuous fasting, it's best to originally change to some low-sugar, high-sound fat eating regime for fourteen days. This will make it possible for the body to become familiar with using fat instead of sugar as a wellspring of energy. That suggests getting off, everything being equal, grains (bread, snacks, baked goods, rice, pasta), vegetables, and processed vegetable oils. This may limit most symptoms associated with fasting.

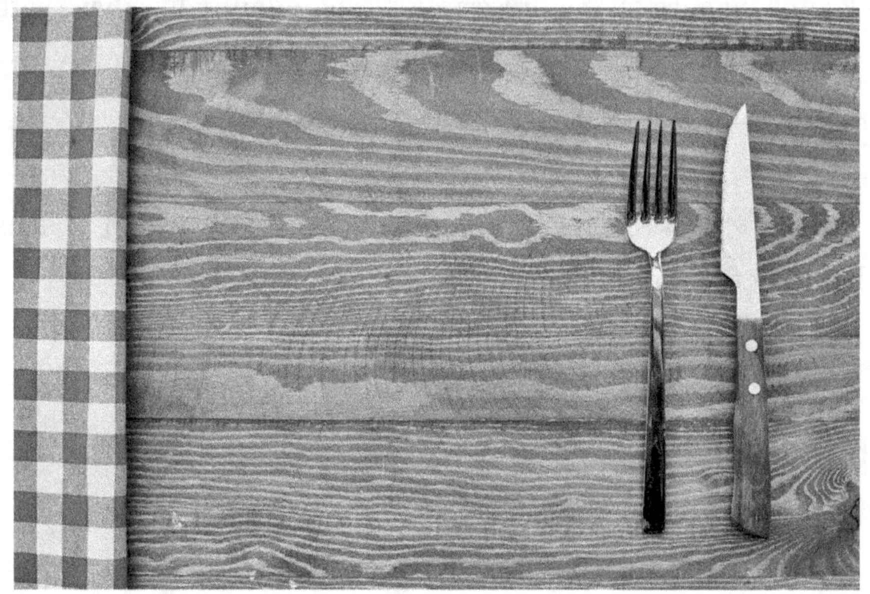

CHAPTER TWO
TYPES OF INTERMITTENT FASTING AND BENEFITS

There are a couple of different procedures for performing discontinuous fasting -- most of which include things like parting daily or weekly to fasting and eating intervals.

The fasting period: you consume next to nothing.

All these would be very well-known approaches:

• The 16/8 plan: Also known as the lean gain's tradition, involves skipping breakfast and restricting your day daily eating interval to 8 hours, by way of instance, 1--9 p.m. Now you fast for 16 hours at the center.

• Eat-Stop-Eat: Including fasting for 24 hours, even more than once each week, for example by not needing from dinner daily before dinner the next day.

• The 5:2 eating regularly: With these strategies, you consume only 500--600 calories on two non-sequential times of this week, nevertheless, eat the other five days.

By lessening your calorie entrance, these techniques must lead to weight loss if you do not repay by ingesting considerably more during the ingestion time frames.

Numerous individuals find the 16/8 approach is the least complicated, typically maintainable and simplest to stick to. It is also very mainstream.

Outlined are a couple of unique approaches to performing discontinuous fasting. Each of them divides the week or week into fasting and eating intervals.
How it affects your cells and hormones

At the stage when you fast, a few things happen in your own body on the mobile and nuclear levels.

For example, your body changes hormone levels to create burn muscle versus fat progressively offered.

Your cells also start significant repair procedures and adjust the outflow of attributes.

Here are a couple of changes that occur in your body if you fast:

• Human Growth Hormone (HGH): The levels of growth hormone soar, expanding up to 5-overlay. This has advantages for fat loss misfortune and muscle gain, to provide a few examples.

• Insulin: Insulin efficiency is enhanced and amounts of insulin fall radically. Reduced insulin levels make muscle to fat ratio to be progressively enhanced.

• Cellular fix: Once fasted, your cells begin cell repair forms. This comprises autophagy, where cells process and expel useless and old proteins with the advancement of cells inside.

• Gene articulation: You can find changes at the capacity of attributes diagnosed with lifetime and confidence from illness.

All these alterations in hormone levels, mobile capacity, and excellent articulation are liable for the health care benefits of intermittent fasting.

Outline: When you fast, human growth hormone levels go up and insulin levels return. Your body's cells also alter the announcement of attributes and begin substantial cell repair forms.

It's an extremely successful weight loss tool.

Weight reduction is the most frequently recognized explanation behind people to try intermittent fasting. By causing you to cat fewer suppers, intermittent fasting may prompt a programmed reduction in calorie entrance.

Furthermore, discontinuous fasting affects hormone levels to promote weight loss.

Notwithstanding bringing insulin down and enlarging growth hormone levels, it assembles the coming of the fat intensive hormone norepinephrine (noradrenaline).

On account of those alterations in hormones, transient fasting can enlarge your metabolic rate by 3.6--14 percent.

By assisting you to eat less and eat more calories, intermittent fasting induces weight reduction by altering the 2 sides of their calorie condition.

Studies show that discontinuous fasting may be an incredibly miraculous weight reduction device.

A 2014 research study found this ingestion example may result in 3--8 percent weight loss over 3--24 weeks, and it is a remarkable amount, compared with most weight-loss beliefs.

In a similar report, people also lost 4--7 percent of the midriff perimeter, demonstrating a remarkable loss of dangerous gut fat which develops around your organs and triggers the disease.

Another research suggested that discontinuous fasting induces less muscle misfortune compared to the standard method of persistent calorie confinement.

In any case, do not forget that the principal reason for its abundance is that intermittent fasting induces you to consume fewer calories. In case you gorge and consume massive sums throughout your eating intervals, you might not lose any weight at all.

Rundown intermittent fasting can marginally encourage digestion while assisting you to consume fewer calories. It is an exceptionally strong approach to lose weight and belly fat.

There are diverse intermittent fasting methods. All these are:

• 5:2: This approach allows you to consume typically five times each week. The other two days will be the fasting times, although you do even now eat. Just keep it somewhere in the assortment of 500 and 600 calories.

• Eat-stop-eat: With this, you limit all nutrition for 24 hours, even more than once each week.

• 16/8: You consume the entirety of your own day daily calories within an abbreviated period -- normally 6 to 8 hours and fast for your remaining 14 to 16 hours. You can do this frequently, or a few times per week.

• Bulletproof irregular fasting most carefully takes following the 16/8 plan, yet with a single essential comparison: you drink a few Bulletproof Coffee at the very first portion of the day. It is a wise hack to maintain the cravings for food while continuing to fast. Whatever the case, more about this later.

Medical benefits of discontinuous fasting

At this stage, if you don't consume any nourishment to get a set timeframe daily, you do your own body and your brain a great mess. It is well appropriate from a developmental angle. For a long time in history, folks were not ingesting three nourishing dinners every day, along with brushing on bites. Instead, folks developed in situations where there was not a great deal of nourishment, and they figured out the way to thrive when fasting. Nowadays, we do not have to pursue nutrition (even though pursuing your own meat is anything but an ill-conceived idea!). Or perhaps we undergo a sizable part of our times prior to PCs, and we consume at whatever stage we desire -- although our bodies are not adjusted to this behavior.

Shifting into a discontinuous fasting diet develops the points of confinement and lifts your display in a variety of ways. Listed below are a part of the extraordinary benefits of intermittent fasting:

• Encourages weight loss

• Increases vitality

• Promotes cell repair and autophagy (if your own body expends faulty tissue in order to make new components)

• reduces insulin resistance and guarantees against type 2 diabetes

• Lowers terrible cholesterol

• interrupts life length

• shield against neurodegenerative Maladies, e.g. Alzheimer's and Parkinson's

• Improves lifts and memory mind work

• Makes cells more powerful

Numerous studies are performed on intermittent fasting, at the 2 animals and people.

All these examinations have shown that it may have revolutionary advantages for weight reduction and the health of their own bodies and mind. It may even help you with living more.

Here are the key medical benefits of discontinuous fasting:

• Weight Hazards: As referenced previously, discontinuous fasting can help you with becoming healthier and paunch fat, without needing to limit calories (1, 13 trusted source) intentionally.

• Insulin barrier: Irregular fasting may diminish insulin resistance, bringing down sugar --6 percent and fasting insulin levels by 20--31 percent, which should guarantee against type 2 diabetes.

• Inflammation: Several assessments show decreases in markers of aggravation, an integral driver of many incessant infections.

• Heart health: Intermittent fasting may reduce "awful" LDL cholesterol, blood glucose, incendiary markers, sugar, and insulin obstruction -- most of the risk factors for coronary disease.

• Cancer: Animal analyses suggest that intermittent fasting can expect malignant growth.

• Brain health: Intermittent fasting increases the cerebrum hormone BDNF and might assist the growth of new cells. It may likewise guarantee against Alzheimer's illness.

• Anti-maturing: Irregular fasting can extend life expectancy. Studies have shown that fasting rodents dwelt 36--83% more.

Recall that mining is still in its start phases. A high number of those investigations were small, current or contributive in animals. Quite a few inquiries currently can not appear to get answered in more outstanding human tests.

Rundown intermittent fasting may have numerous benefits for your entire body and cerebrum. It can induce weight reduction and might reduce your threat of type 2 diabetes, coronary disease, and disorder. It may likewise help you with living longer.

Makes your healthy lifestyle simpler

Eating nicely is simple, yet it very well might be incredibly tough to maintain.

One of the principal impediments is all the work necessary to prepare for and cook strong suppers.

Irregular fasting can make matters easier since you do not need to plan, cook, or keep eating the exact same dinners.

Hence, discontinuous fasting is known among the life-hacking swarm, as it enhances your health while at precisely the exact same time streamlining your daily life concurrently.

Synopsis: Among the substantial benefits of discontinuous fasting is that it makes intelligent dieting simpler. You will find fewer dinners you need to strategize, concoct and wash afterward.
Who must perform or avoid it?

Irregular fasting is not for everyone.

If you are underweight or possess a background marked with dietary difficulties, you shouldn't fast without counseling with health proficient first.

These scenarios very well might be out and otherwise harmful.

If girls quickly?

There is some evidence that intermittent fasting might not be as beneficial for women, all things considered for guys.

For example, one examination demonstrated it enhanced insulin efficiency in men but declined sugar control in women.

Even though human analyses at this stage are inaccessible, examinations in rodents reveal that intermittent fasting may cause female rodents anorexic, masculinized, barren, and lead them to overlook cycles.

There are various story reports of women whose menstrual period stopped when they started doing IF and returned into normal if they continued with their previous eating style.

Thus, women should be more careful with intermittent fasting.

They should pursue distinct rules, like slipping to the practice and stopping immediately on the off possibility they have any problems such as amenorrhea (nonappearance of the female cycle).

The off probability, you have problems with ripeness too as are trying to envision, think about holding off irregular fasting for now. This eating style is probably likewise an ill-conceived notion in the event you're pregnant or breastfeeding.

Rundown individuals that are underweight or have a history of dietary issues shouldn't fast. There's also some evidence that intermittent fasting may be dangerous to certain women.

Safety and Negative Effects

Yearning is the principal response of discontinuous fasting.

You may likewise feel weak and your cerebrum might not function as you are used to.

This may only be impermanent since it could put aside some attempt for the body to adapt to the new feast program.

The off probability, you have an ailment, you need to seek advice with your primary care doctor before trying irregular fasting.

This is especially important in case you

• Have diabetes.

• suffer from sugar rule.

• Have a low heartbeat.

• On medication.

• Are underweight.

• Have a past full of dietary issues.

• Are a woman who's trying to imagine.

• Are a woman with a past full of amenorrhea.

• Are pregnant or breastfeeding.

Discontinuous fasting includes a remarkable health profile. There's nothing insecure about not eating for a while in the event you're strong and well-supported generally.

Synopsis: the most frequently recognized manifestation of discontinuous fasting is appetite. People with specific ailments shouldn't fast without counseling with a professional first.

Starting

Odds are that you have only done numerous intermittent fasts during your lifetime.

On the off probability that you have at any stage had dinner; at the point dozed late rather than had occurred before lunch the next day; at the point, you have presumably as of today fasted for 16+ hours.

A couple of individuals intuitively consume this way. They essentially do not feel hungry during the first period of the day.

Numerous people consider the 16/8 plan the least challenging and most economical way of discontinuous fasting -- you need to try this practice first.

In the event that you believe its easy, and feel good throughout the period; at this point possibly give transferring a shot to additionally grown fasts like 24-hour fasts 1--2 times per week (Eat-Stop-Eat) or simply eating 500--600 calories 1--2 days out of every week (5:2 eating regular).

Another methodology is to simply quit at whatever stage it is advantageous -- basically skip suppers again and when you are not eager or do not have the chance to cook.

There is no persuasive reason to pursue a coordinated intermittent fasting plan to recognize probably some of the benefits.

Diagnosis: Together with several methodologies, find something which you enjoy and can accommodate your schedule.

Rundown: it is prescribed to start with this 16/8 plan at this point, and possibly later proceed ahead to more fasts. It is crucial to try and find a plan that is appropriate for you.

Kinds OF INTERMITTENT FASTING:

Irregular fasting comes in various structures and each might have a specific arrangement of one of some kind advantages. Each kind of discontinuous fasting was formed from the fasting-to-eating percentage. The benefits and adequacy of the several conventions may compare on a single assumption and it's essential to determine which one is most appropriate for you. Factors that can influence which to select include wellness goals, daily plan/schedule, and present wellbeing status. The most frequently recognized forms of IF are day fasting, time-limited strengthening, and transformed fasting.

1. Interchange day fasting:

This methodology includes substituting extended spans of certainly no calories (from nutrition or refreshment) with long stretches of complimentary promoting and ingesting whatever you would like.

This arrangement has appeared to aid weight loss, improve blood glucose and triglyceride (fat) levels, and enhance annoyance markers for elimination from the blood.

The basic ruin with such intermittent fasting is it is by far the most difficult to remain with because of this demonstrated craving during fasting times.

2. Adjusted fasting - 5:2 diet

Adjusted fasting is a tradition with altered fasting days, no matter how the fasting times consider some nourishment entrance. By and large 20-25percent of average calories can be consumed on fasting times; therefore, in case you normally consume 2000 calories on normal eating times, then you'd be allowed 400-500 calories on fasting times. The 5:2 part of the eating regime alludes to the ratio of non-fasting to flaxseed times. So, on this regular, you'd consume normally for 5 continuous days in the point fast or restrict calories to 20-25percent for two back to back days.

This convention is amazing for weight loss, body business, and might likewise gain the rule of sugar, lipids, and aggravation. Studies have shown the 5:2 seminar to be effective for weight loss, improve/lower annoyance markers in the bloodstream (3), and provide indications drifting updates in insulin resistance. In animal experiments, this altered flaxseed 5:2 eating regimen caused diminished fat, diminished craving hormones (leptin), and enlarged amounts of a protein accountable for improvements in fat intensive and sugar principle (adiponectin).

The modified 5:2 fasting convention isn't anything but hard to pursue and contains few negative symptoms that comprised yearning, low energy, and a few crabbiness when beginning the application. Rather than in any instance, contemplates have noted improvements, by way of instance, diminished stress, less outrage, less fatigue, updates in fearlessness, and an increasingly positive mood.

3. TIME-RESTRICTED FEEDING:

In case you know anyone that has stated that they do discontinuous fasting, the odds are it's as time-limited sustaining. This is a sort of discontinuous fasting that's used daily and it features just devouring calories through just a bit daily' and fasting for the remainder of. Daily fasting interims at time-confined strengthening may stretch from 12-20 hours, using the most frequently recognized approach being 16/8 (fasting for 16 hours, devouring calories for 2). With this convention, the hour daily is not important so long as you're fasting for a back to backstage and eating on your allowed timespan. For example, on a 16/8 time-limited nourishing job. one person may consume their very first dinner at 7 AM and final feast at 3 PM (fast from 3 PM-7 AM), while someone else could consume their dinner at 1 PM and continue dinner at 9 PM (fast from 9 PM-1 PM). This tradition is meant to be performed daily over substantial stretches of time and can be completely flexible so long as you're staying within the fasting/eating window(s).

Time-restricted encouragement is among the simplest to pursue methods for discontinuous fasting. Using this together with your everyday work and remainder calendar might help achieve ideal metabolic power. Time-limited strengthening is an outstanding program to pursue weight loss and body construction enhancements as some additional by and large health benefits. The few human preliminaries which were led noted enormous decreases in fat, decreases in blood sugar, and improvements in cholesterol with no progressions in stress, sorrow, outrage, fatigue, or disarray. Another basic result from animal tests suggested time-restricted sustaining to safeguard against corpulence, higher insulin levels, fatty liver disease, and aggravation.

The simple program and promising effects of time-confined encouraging may allow it to be an unbelievable alternative for weight loss and ceaseless illness counteractive action across the board. While executing this option, it may be great in the first place with a lesser fasting-to-eating ratio like 12/12 hours and in the very long term stir your way around 16/8 hours.

The fundamental question about intermittent fasting:

Is there some nourishment or refreshment I'm permitted to expend while still on intermittent fasting? Except if you're performing the altered fasting 5:2 eating regimen (referenced above), then do your best not to consume or ingesting anything that contains calories. Water, black espresso, and some other nourishments/drinks which don't include carbs are ok to consume through a fasting period. Truth be told, adequate water entrance is essential throughout IF and a few say that ingesting dark espresso whilst fasting empowers diminishing appetite.

Irregular fasting is now a well-known approach to use for the own body's ordinary fat-consuming capability to shed weight in a brief period. Whatever the case, a lot of people will need to understand how discontinuous fasting operate and just how precisely does this function? At the stage when you go to get an off-beat timeframe without eating, your body alters the way it produces compounds and hormones, which can be great for fat disputes. These are the principal fasting benefits and the way they achieve those benefits.

Hormones construct the assumption of metabolic capabilities including the pace at which you have fat. The development hormone is made by your own body and progress the breakdown of fat from the body to provide energy. At the stage when you fast for some time, your body starts to expand its growth hormone production. Likewise, fasting tries to reduce the amount of insulin within the circulatory system, assuring your body absorbs fat rather than putting it away.

A momentary fast that keeps moving 12-72 hours increases the digestion and adrenaline levels, which makes you increase the number of calories consumed daily. Moreover, those who fast likewise achieve more outstanding vitality through enlarged adrenaline, forcing them not to feel tired although they aren't getting calories by and large. Regardless of how you might feel like, fasting ought to bring about diminished energy, the body makes up for this, assuring a fatty consuming method.

A great many men and women who consume every 3-5 hours basically eat sugar instead of fat. Fasting for longer intervals makes your digestion to swallow fat. Ahead of the conclusion of a 24-hour fast day, your body has spent glycogen stores in the very first few hours and has spent approximately 18 of the hour's intensive fat stores in the body. For any person who's routinely lively, and yet at precisely the exact same time struggles with fat misfortune, discontinuous fasting may construct fat misfortune without inclining an exercise program or correct an eating regime program.

Another benefit of discontinuous fasting is that it essentially resets somebody's body. Opting to go a day or so without ingesting affects an individual's cravings, which makes them feel excited after a time. On the off probability that you struggle with consistently needing nutrition, intermittent fasting may empower your body to adapt to occasions of not eating and help you not to feel hungry constantly. Quite a few people see they begin to consume more valuable and progressively controlled eating regimens whenever they fast irregularly for one day in seven days.

Discontinuous fasting changes, however, are by and large suggested for approximately one day consistently. On this day, a person might have a fluid supplement packed smoothie or a low-calorie alternative. Since the body changes using an intermittent fasting strategy, this is normally not important. Discontinuous fasting reduces fat shops normally from the body, by simply altering the digestion to different fat rather than muscle or sugar. It's been used by many people viably and it's an easy technique to roll out an improvement that is beneficial. For any person who struggles with stubborn fat and can be worn out on habitual abstinence from excessive food intake, intermittent fasting provides a very simple and productive option for fat misfortune and a more advantageous method of life.

Intermittent fasting: A powerful tool for weight loss and diabetes control

A matter of primary importance, fasting is not starvation. Starvation is the automated forbearance from restricted ingestion due to external powers; this happens in the middle of starvation and war when nutrition is infrequent. Fasting, on the other hand, is deliberate, informed, and regulated. Nourishment is immediately available, yet we decide to not consume it due to otherworldly, health, or various explanations.

Fasting is as old as humans, a lot more experienced than various other kinds of diets. Old civic institutions, very similar to the Greeks, believed there was something inherently valuable to intermittent fasting. They have been frequently called events of recovering, purging, cleaning, or detoxification. For all intents and purposes, every civilization and faith in the world practice a couple of sculptures of fasting.

Ahead to the visual appeal of agribusiness, individuals never ate three suppers daily as well as nibbling at the center. We ate only when we found nourishment that could be days or hours separated. Consequently, in the improvement perspective, eating three suppers daily is not a necessity for endurance. We wouldn't have left due to a creature category.

Fast forward into the 21st century, we've got this antiquated practice gradually dismissed. After all, fasting is completely dreadful for the company! Nourishment manufacturers urge us to consume a lot of suppers and snacks per day. Medical specialists caution that preventing dinner alone will have dire wellbeing outcomes. With time, these messages are so well-bored to our minds.

Fasting has no standard term. It may be achieved for a few hours to numerous times to weeks end. Irregular fasting is also an eating plan where we cycle one of fasting and ordinary eating. Shorter fasts of 16-20 hours are generally accomplished even much more of their moment, even daily. Longer fasts, often 24-36 hours, are completed 2-3 times per week. As it happens, we have a complete daily fast for a period of 12 hours or so, one of breakfast and dinner.

Fasting has been completed by a massive number of people for a massive number of years. Is it unfortunate? No. Truly, various investigations have suggested that it has enormous medical benefits.

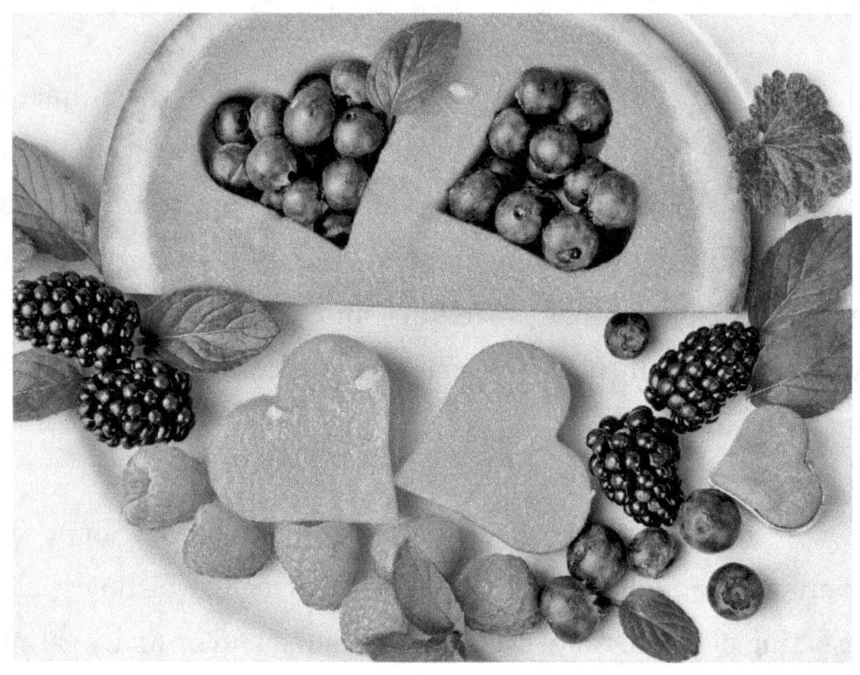

CHAPTER THREE
COMMON MISTAKES TO AVOID

With a growing amount of people in the world fighting to get healthier, it is no huge surprise there prevailing trends of eating fewer carbohydrates that are popularized through the overriding press.

As signaled from the WHO, approximately 52 percent of the entire population is either obese or corpulent. A high number of those individuals have tried to get fit in any event earlier or later in their own lives, and a few have tried different items with outrageous eating of fewer carbohydrates followed by the fad absorption of fewer calories.

For instance, as the study seems, an outrageous weight reduction diet is not only ineffectual as a very long-haul arrangement, but it very well might be unbelievably harming for your wellbeing.
Outstanding eating of less junk food prompts muscle wasting

Outstanding weight-loss abstinence from food, for the most part, comprise serious calorie restriction with the purpose of shedding a great deal of weight in the shortest amount of period possible. While those ingestion regimens will automatically prompt unbelievable weight reduction within the first barely few weeks, then you need to bear in mind that you risked losing muscle tissue until you discover the chance to shed weight.

As indicated by medicinal experts, eccentric abstaining from excess food consumption will initially prompt water weight loss, at the point of muscular decay, as well as fat hardship. Scientist G.L. Thorpe has explained this quite some time back, expressing that our body does not especially absorb fat when we eat less. It instead, squanders all the body tissues, such as the bones and muscles.
Muscle wasting interrupts your digestion.

The motivation behind why your system aims muscle tissue when you're starving yourself is because it aims to safeguard vitality when nutrition is insufficient. To explain this further -- your system requires additional energy in order to maintain muscle tissue than it will, in order to care for fat.

When there is a lack of energy from nutrition as in cases of absurd eating of junk food, your body will attempt to evacuate among the human body's most noteworthy energy shoppers -- the muscles.

This will occur no matter if you're doing weight reduction clinics you might believe help reconstruct more muscle. Be as it may, the terrible news does not end there.

Recall that lost mass prompts a lower basal metabolic rate, and a reduced metabolic rate inspires you to have more weight reduction. These realities explain why such a high number of people go through the jo-jo effect after an outrageous eating pattern.

A study spread in the Journals of Gerontology found that the calorie restriction decreases vitality expenditure. What this means is that being on a remarkably low-carb diet can prompt more slow digestion which makes future weight-loss problematic if not certainly impossible.

Moreover, slims down which are low in carbs are often restrictive and everything considered, unfit to tackle your body's problems for basic nutritional supplements. Therefore, being on the condition, an 800-calorie diet plan is most likely going to prompt nutritional supplement lack that can damage your wellbeing.

A concentrate that has been dispersed at the Journal of the International Society of Sports Nutrition scrutinized the pervasiveness of micronutrient inadequacies in widespread slims down, and the results were striking.

The evaluation discovered a restrictive weight reduction diet known as the best lifestyle diet fulfilled just 55 percent of daily micronutrient requirements while the exceptionally famous South beach diet fulfilled just 22 percent of their day daily prerequisites for micronutrients. Other negative outcomes are fewer carbohydrates, as well as restrictive weight reduction programs, include osteoporosis, obesity, discouragement, kidney stones, and in extreme instances scurvy if the eating regimen is insufficient in nutrient C.

The best way to get in shape right?

For one thing, you need to bear in mind that successful weight loss consistently goes forward bit by a little bit. This means changing to some wise dieting propensity which is possible to pursue for a substantial amount of time to come as practicing a week per week assumption.

You should additionally consume fewer calories than you personally, as a guideline reach for weight loss to happen. As indicated by means of an examination distributed previously from the Journal of Research in Medical Sciences, devouring fewer calories would be the ideal weight reduction program, especially when combined with low-GI and moderate fat intake. Just make sure that you reduce your calorie entrance by 300-500 calories as indicated by Harvard Health Publications.

For example, if your typical eating regimen comprises of 2500 calories, then begin eating 2200 calories. Your body will put aside the attempt to modify in accordance with this discreet caloric shortfall, yet earlier or later, you can shed a few calories.

Just make sure you don't eat everywhere under 1200 on the off possibility that you're a woman or below 1500 on the off probability that you're a guy to steer clear of micronutrient lacks. Various items to help you with becoming thinner include discovering daily weight-loss inspiration pointers to help prop you up and assessing your health along with your primary care doctor to assess whether fundamental wellbeing requirements are slowing down your weight loss.

Diets do not do the job, yet superior dieting does

Instead of following prevailing fad diet drifts which you see being advanced with lean renowned men and women, nutritionists would advise that you pursue decent dieting.

By switching to smart dieting instead of a low-carb diet that does not work, you will have the choice to shed weight slowly and address your body's problems for essential nutrients.

At this stage, as soon as your body is solid, and your penis is well-supported, you're certain to experience effective long drag weight loss. Another motive behind this is really that intelligent dieting is a good deal easier to stick to over the long haul when compared with unthinkable and restrictive eating regimens.

As per a passing dispersed in the Journal of Food and Nutrition, switching to smart dieting involves creating an enormous way of lifestyle changes, focusing on nutrition quality, and correcting your own nutrients.

A similar section documents the health benefits of fantastic dieting that include the diminished threat of cardiovascular disease, diabetes, malignancy and of course, a better body structure.

Easily Disregard Immediate Weight Loss

You may hear reports of people losing a huge amount of burden by following inconceivable eating regimens. These reports are standard elements of boosting attempts for weight reduction products and abstaining from excess food consumption novels which are conceivably hindering health. Sticking to shown actualities is your principal way possible to get fit efficiently and safely.

Weight reduction requires that you cut down on your calories bit by bit without undermining your health. Additionally, it includes regular exercise to enlarge energy use and to fabricate more muscular tissue.
What is the best diet to get audio weight loss?

Get any eating regular publication and it'll profess to maintain each of the answers to efficiently losing all the weight that you want --and keeping it off. Some propose the secret is to consume less and exercise; others that reduce fat is the ideal thing to do, but others endorse eliminating carbs. Overall, what could be a fantastic idea for you to take?

The fact of the matter is that there isn't anyone size fits all" response for endless sound weight loss. What works for one person might not work for you, because our bodies respond distinctively to different nourishments, contingent upon hereditary attributes as well as other health facets. To find the strategy for weight loss that's right for you may probably need substantial investment and need commitment, dedication, and some experimentation with numerous nourishments and diets.

Even though a couple of men and women respond well to tallying calories or relative restrictive methods, others respond better to get more chances in organizing their get-healthy plans. Being allowed to only maintain a strategic space from singed nourishments or cut back on refined carbohydrates can place them up for advancement. Do not get too disheartened if an eating regimen that worked for one more individual does not do the job for you. In addition, don't pummel yourself whether an eating regimen that you stay with proves unreasonably prohibitive. Invariably, an eating regimen is right for you if it is one you're able to remain with for some time.

Maintain in your mind: while there is no easy remedy to losing weight, there is a lot of steps that you can take to develop a more favorable institution with nourishment, restrain passionate causes to gorging, and achieve a good weight.

Two notable weight-loss systems

1. Cut calories

A few experts accept that efficiently coping with your weight boils down to some simple requirement: If you consume fewer calories than you eat, you get slimmer. Sounds easy, is not that so? At that stage, why is shedding fat so challenging?

• Weight misfortune is certifiably not a straight event after some time. At that stage, once you cut calories, you might shed weight for the very first few weeks, for example, and then something changes. You consume a comparable number of calories; nevertheless, you lose less weight or no fat anyway. That's about the grounds that if you get healthier you are losing water and slim tissue equally as fat; then your digestion alleviates back, along with your own body changes in various ways. Along those lines, in order to keep losing weight weekly, you need to keep cutting off calories.

• A calorie is not always a calorie. Eating 100 calories of high fructose corn syrup, for example, can otherwise affect your entire body than eating 100 calories. The stunt for continuing weight reduction would be to ditch the nourishments which are pressed with carbs but do not cause you to feel complete (like snacks) and supplant them with nourishments which shirt you off without even being piled with calories (such as vegetables).

• a lot of us don't generally consume only to meet hunger. We likewise visit nutrition for relaxation or to calm stress --that can quickly crash any weight reduction program.

2. Cut carbohydrates

An alternative way of review weight reduction modulates the problem as none of devouring such a high number of calories, but rather the way your system amasses fat following to expending sugars--especially the task of the hormone insulin. At the stage when you consume a dinner, then starches in the nutrition enter your circulatory system as sugar. In order to maintain your sugar levels under wraps, then your body regularly consumes this off sugar before it absorbs fat out of a feast.

Maintaining a fantastic wellness

Everybody needs to be strong; however, not a lot of jobs to go the extra mile and adopt a solid propensity on a regular assumption. Whatever the instance, with much more mindfulness towards a healthy and sound means of life, folks increasingly are going in the path of it. The way to maintaining good wellbeing is the combination of numerous elements like regular exercise, excellent eating routine, stress the plank, work-life balance, audio relations, higher assurance, and that is just the tip of this iceberg. Nothing could be substituted for another. In case you're looking for some vital guidelines on the most skillful process to maintain up great health, measure along these lines.

1. Stay hydrated

How to maintain up great health? It is as simple as drinking heaps of water and fluids to keep yourself hydrated regularly. Drinking water generally during this time is essential because we keep losing water out of our own body as urine and sweat. Water does some major capacities, as an instance; flushing germs from your liver, assisting absorption, distributing nutritional supplements and oxygen into the cells, preventing stoppage and maintaining up the electrolyte (sodium) equilibrium.

2. Eat lots of fruits and vegetables

The body demands a constant inflow of minerals and nutrients. An eating regimen rich in leafy foods ensures that your body receives each of the supplements needed. All leafy foods have their own effect on providing different minerals and nutrients. Contain a whole lot of splendid and deep-hued veggies and organic products such as apples, red berries, purple berries, and lush greens since they are wealthy in cancer prevention agents that fight illness-causing free radicals. You prepare a few interesting plates of mixed greens, or perhaps make a yummy organic merchandise chaat or blend them into thick smoothies.

3. Do not limit your meals

Every supper has its own impact. Afterward, skirting among those 3 important dinners of this day may have a negative impact. Your cerebrum and body need fuel to operate. Your brain wants a stockpile of sugar and a lack of it can cause you to get torpid. Skipping suppers can make your digestion down, and this may prompt weight gain or make it more challenging to get healthier. At the stage when you bypass dishes, your body turns on the 'endurance style', which basically implies it succeeds for much more nutrition than anticipated, which finally contributes to pigging out.

4. Prevent fatty, processed foods

The fresher, the better. Affordable food and ready or bundled nutrition often follow various additives and additional substances to enlarge rack live. Furthermore, they may hide substantial levels of sodium and sugar which may construct the threat of life infections like diabetes, hypertension, circulatory stress, heftiness, and the sky is the limit from there. Handled nourishments also have 'satisfying' quality that suggests that for their succulent, sweet or zesty flavor, your head starts thinking about them as remunerating nourishments that arouses superfluous yearnings.

5. Contain more lean meats, low-fat dairy products, and whole grains for your diet

The way to maintain good wellbeing is to get a decent eating regimen with meals grown on the floor. You want a decent mix of milk, milk products, meat, legumes, and vegetables. Select low-fat milk, yogurt, cheddar, lean beef, fish (cut on reading beef), darker rice, millets and oats to get much more favorable outcomes. With respect to grains, whole grains tend to be better. Processed bread and grains such as Maida and white rice saturated in nutritional supplements. Whole grains are piled with fiber and nutritional supplements which keep you full and satisfied; It also comprises of stock Health Practitioner and Macrobiotic Nutritionist Shilpa Arora. The type of starches you eat is important. A huge part of our starches should be low levels which suggest that they should not result in rapid spikes on your sugar levels and provide moderate birth of energy." Whole grains, dals, rajma and vegetables - these are phenomenal wellsprings of unpredictable and very low GI sugars.

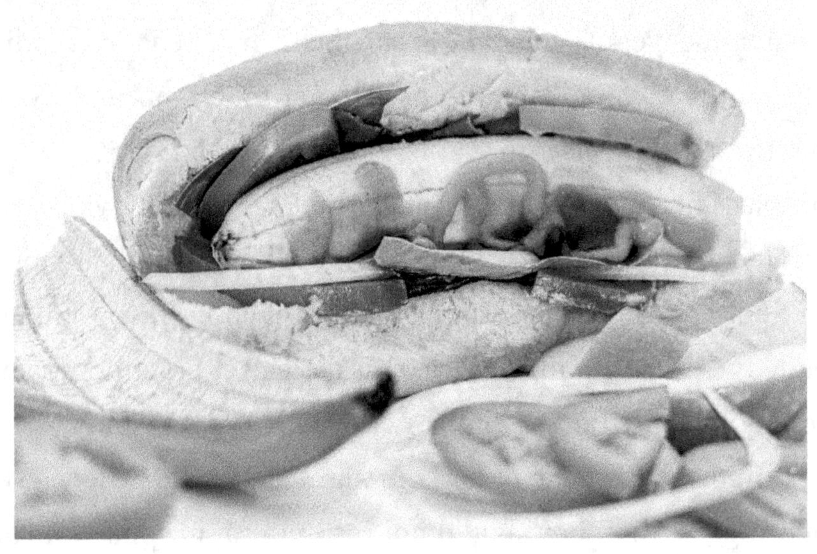

CHAPTER FOUR
BENEFITS OF INTERMITTENT FASTING FOR WOMEN

What Happens When We Eat Consistently?

Ahead to entering the benefits of intermittent fasting, it's best to understand why eating 5-6 meals every day or at frequent periods (the cautious inverse of fasting) can attain more harm than anything else.

At this stage, we consume nutrition energy. The vital hormone contained is insulin (delivered from the pancreas), which ascends during suppers. The 2 protein and sugars. Fat activates a little more insulin effect; nevertheless, fat is in a while consumed alone.

Insulin has two important capacities -

• First, it enables your system to immediately begin using nutrition energy. Starches are rapidly changed over into sugar, thus increasing glucose levels. Insulin guides glucose to the body tissues to be used as energy. Proteins are split into amino acids and overabundance amino acids may be converted into sugar.

Protein does not actually raise blood sugar, yet it may rekindle insulin. Fats have a negligible effect on insulin.

• Secondly, insulin shops away overabundance energy for some time afterward. Insulin converts overabundance sugar into glycogen and keeps it in the liver. Whatever the situation, there's a breaking point to just how a great deal of glycogen could be placed away. When the point is come to, the liver starts shifting sugar into fat. The fat is then cared for at the liver (in overabundance, it will become fatty liver) or fat stores in the body (often put away as Energetic or gut fat).

In this manner, once we consume and simmer for the whole period of the day, we're constantly in a nourished condition and insulin levels remain high. Therefore, we're spending most of the day setting away nutrition energy.

What Happens When We Quickly?

The way toward using and putting nourishment away into energy that occurs when we consume goes backward once we fast. Insulin levels fall, inciting the entire body to start consuming place away energy. Glycogen, the sugar that's put away from the liver, is gotten to and used. From this point forward, the body starts to separate place away muscle to fat ratio for energy.

Together with those traces, the body basically exists in two countries - the fed country with higher insulin along with the fasting condition with reduced insulin. We're either setting away nourishment energy or we're consuming nutrition energy. On the off chance that fasting and eating are corrected, at this point, there isn't any weight gain. In case we spend much of the day eating and setting energy away, there's a good likelihood that in due time, we might end up putting on weight.

Irregular Fasting Versus Constant Calorie-Restriction

The little control methodology of metabolic reduction is the most frequently recognized dietary tip for weight loss and type two diabetes. As an example, the American Diabetes Association prescribes a 500-750 kcal/day energy shortage together with standard bodily motion. Dietitians pursue this strategy and indicate eating 4-6 small suppers for the whole period of this day.

Can the little control process work within the long haul? Seldom. An accomplice study using a 9-year follow-up by the UK on 176,495 obese people revealed that only 3,528 of these prevail with respect to attaining ordinary bodyweight, until the conclusion of this exam. That's a disappointment rate of 98 percent!

Irregular fasting is not consistent with caloric confinement. Limiting calories triggers a compensatory increment in yearning and much more dreadful, a diminishing from the human body's metabolic rate, a twofold revile! Since when we're consuming fewer calories every single day, it ends up becoming progressively more difficult to get fit and also a good deal easier to recuperate weight after we've lost it. This form of diet puts your system into a "starvation mode" as digestion flames upward down to conserve energy.

Discontinuous fasting does not have one of these advantages.

Medical Benefits of Irregular Fasting

It builds digestion and encourages fat and muscle versus fat misfortune.

Perhaps not at all like a daily caloric reduction diet, discontinuous fasting increases digestion. This bodes well from an endurance perspective. On the off possibility that we do not consume, the body uses put away energy as fuel, together with the aim that we're able to stay living to detect another feast. Hormones permit the body to change vitality resources from nutrition to muscle.

Studies reveal this miracle clearly. For example, four days of nonstop fasting enlarged the Basal Metabolic rate by 12 percent. Amounts of this synapse norepinephrine, which divides the body for action, enlarged by 117 percent. Unsaturated fats at the flow system enlarged over 370 percent as the body shifted from absorbing nutrition to consuming put away fats.

No misfortune in the majority

Perhaps not whatsoever like a continuous calorie-confinement diet, intermittent fasting does not consume muscles in the same amount of consumption dreaded. In 2010, experts took a gander in a gathering of subjects that underwent 70 days of trade daily fasting (ate a single afternoon and fasted the next). Their majority started at 52.0 kg and ended in 51.9 kg. Therefore, there was no reduction of muscles; nevertheless, they dropped 11.4percent of fat and found substantial updates in LDL cholesterol and triglyceride levels.

Throughout fasting, the body typically generates progressively human growth hormone to safeguard slender bones and muscles. Bulk is often protected till muscle to fat ratio drops under 4 percent. In this manner, the huge majority aren't at risk of muscle-squandering whilst performing discontinuous fasting.

Turn around insulin resistance, type two diabetes, and fatty liver

Sort 2 diabetes is a condition where there's essentially an inordinate quantity of sugar from the body, to the point that the mobiles can not react to insulin and consume any more sugar in the bloodstream (insulin obstruction), causing large glucose. Furthermore, the liver becomes piled with fat since it tries to eliminate the prosperity sugar by altering it over and putting it away.

Subsequently, to reverse this ailment, two things will need to happen

• First, stop putting sugar into the entire body.

• Second, eat the rest of the sugar off.

The finest diet to do this is really a low-sugar, moderate-protein, also high-solid fat eating regime similarly called ketogenetic diet plan. (Remember that starch increases sugar the most, protein marginally, and fat at the least.) That's the reason why a low-carb diet can help decrease the burden of glucose. For certain people, this is because one day is enough to change insulin resistance and type two diabetes. Be as it may, in acute scenarios, diet alone is not adequate.

Shouldn't something be said about exercise? Exercise can help ignite with offing sugar in the skeletal tissues; nevertheless, not all those cells and organs; for instance, greasy liver. Evidently, the clinic is important, yet to extract the prosperity sugar in the organs, there's the requirement to "starve" cells.

Irregular fasting can attain this. That's the motive verifiably; people referred to fasting psychologists or even detox. It tends to be a wonderful asset to eliminate this substantial variety of overabundances. It's the fastest method to reduce blood sugar and insulin levels, and ultimately shifting insulin resistance, type two diabetes, and fatty liver.

Coincidentally, taking insulin for type 2 diabetes does not deal with the most important driver of the matter, which can be overabundance sugar within the body. The facts show that insulin will induce away the glucose in the bloodstream, bringing about reduced blood sugar, yet where can the sugar move? The liver is going to change everything into fat in the liver and fat from the mid-region. Patients that go on insulin often end up putting on more fat, which reduces their diabetes.

Upgrades heart health

In the course of time, higher blood sugar from type two diabetes may damage the nerves and veins which control the center. The more one has diabetes, the greater the chances that coronary disease will be created. By bringing down sugar through discontinuous fasting, the threat of cardiovascular disease and stroke is similarly diminished.

Moreover, discontinuous fasting appeared to enhance cardiovascular strain, aggregate and LDL (awful) cholesterol, blood glucose, and incendiary markers associated with numerous ceaseless ailments.

Lifts intellectual art

Numerous studies revealed fasting has many neurologic benefits including center and consideration, reaction time, instantaneous memory, discernment, and the era of new synapses. Mice ponders also indicated that discontinuous fasting reduces cerebrum annoyance and avoids the unwanted effects of Alzheimer's disease.

What is in the shop with occasional fasting?

Glucose does not crash.

Now and then folks stress that sugar will drop tremendously low through fasting and they'll be unsteady and sweat-soaked. This does not really happen as sugar is strongly observed from the human body and there are assorted tools to keep it at the best possible selection. Through fasting, the body begins to separate glycogen from the liver to release sugar. This occurs each late night during our break.

In case that we fast for more than 24-36 hours, then glycogen stores become emptied and the liver is likely to create new glucose using glycerol that's due to the breakdown of fat (a process known as gluconeogenesis). Besides utilizing sugar, our synapses can similarly use ketones for energy. Ketones are generated when fat is utilized and they're able to provide around 75 percent of the cerebrum's energy requirements (another 25 percent from sugar).

The primary exemption is for the people that are taking diabetic insulin and meds. You must initially advise your primary care doctor as the dosages will probably be diminished as you're fasting. Another thing, on the off probability that you just overmedicate and hypoglycemia results, which is poisonous, you ought to have some sugar to flip around it. This may break the speed and ensure it is counterproductive.

The first light miracle

After a period of fasting, especially toward the start of the day, a couple of men and women experience elevated blood sugar. This afternoon break marvel is an aftereffect of this circadian rhythm whereby just before stimulating, the body exerts considerable levels of a few hormones to prepare for the up and coming day -

• Adrenaline - to provide the body some power

• Growth hormone - to help mend and create fresh protein

• Glucagon - to transfer sugar from the liver into the blood to be used as energy

• Cortisol, the stress hormone - to initiate your system

All these hormones leading to the first portion of the daylight hours, fall to bring down the amounts over the course of the day. In non-diabetics, the degree of the sugar rise is small, and the huge majority will not see it. Be that as it may, for most of the diabetics, there may be a visible spike in blood sugar since the liver dumps sugar to the blood.

This will happen in broadened fasts also. Whenever there's not any nourishment, insulin levels stay low while the liver releases some of its placed away fat and sugar. This is common rather than a terrible thing by any means. The greatness of this spike will diminish since the liver proves to be enlarged with fat and sugar.

Who Shouldn't Do Intermittent Fasting?

• Girls who are pregnant, will be pregnant, or are breastfeeding.

• People that are malnourished or underweight.

• Kids under 18 years of age and older folks.

• People who have gout.

• People who have gastroesophageal celiac disease (GERD).

• People who have dietary issues should initially seek advice with their primary care doctors.

• People that are taking diabetic meds and insulin should originally seek advice with their primary care doctors as dimensions ought to be diminished.

• People that are taking prescriptions should initially seek advice with their primary care doctors as the preparation of medication may be affected.

• People who are feeling pressured or possess cortisol problems shouldn't fast since fasting is just another stressor.

• People that are on exceptionally challenging duties most days of the week shouldn't fast.

How to get ready for irregular fasting?

On the off chance that anyone is considering starting discontinuous fasting, it's best to originally change into some low-sugar, high-sound fat eating regime for three weeks. This will enable the body to become familiar with using fat instead of sugar as a wellspring of energy. That implies disposing of, everything being equal, grains (bread, snacks, baked goods, rice, pasta), vegetables, and processed vegetable oils. This will restrict most symptoms associated with fasting.

Starting from using a briefer rapid of 16 hours; for example, from dinner (8 pm) before lunch (12 pm) the next day. You can eat normally between 12 pm and 8 pm, and you're able to eat a couple of dinners. When you are feeling great with it, then you can stretch out the fast to 18, 20 hours.

For shorter fasts, you can certainly do it every day, consistently. For more extended fasts, by way of instance, 24-36 hours, you can act 1-3 times per week, switching back and forth one of fasting and ordinary ingestion times.

There is not just one single correct fasting routine. There are several, and the secret is to select one which works best for you. A couple of men and women achieve effects with shorter fasts, others might require longer fasts. A couple of folks do a terrific water-tight fast; others do espresso and tea fast, while others a bone reduction fast. Whatever you do, it's critical to stay hydrated and monitor yourself. On the off probability that you are feeling ill anytime, you need to stop straight away. You can be excited; however, you shouldn't feel pumped out.

Weight index is not just about the amount you weigh but additionally mulls on your tallness.

You should realize that your body mass index (BMI) needs to be checked if you are qualified for a medical operation.

The body mass index is the weight in kilograms partitioned from the square foot of your height in yards. You may be qualified if your BMI is greater than 40 (sullen stoutness) or greater than 35 using a real heftiness related health condition, by way of instance, uncontrolled Type 2 diabetes, sleep apnea or intense joint distress that limits your daily exercises.

Recognizing weight reduction dimensions

Using the dimensions of Excess Body Weight (EBW) and Excessive Weight reduction (EWL) motivates us to observe how a great deal of weight loss we should expect that is comparative to our tallness.

You may notice that someone has shed 50 pounds; nevertheless, without discovering their EBW and EWL, there's absolutely no opportunity to get at determining whether they've dropped a ton or even a tiny measure of burden relative with their own body tallness. On the off probability that the person who loses these 50 pounds is significantly taller than you and contains a few pounds more to lose than you, 50 pounds is not that much fat to lose weight. Nonetheless, in the event the person only had 50 pounds to shed, we could affirm that a person who lost 100 percent EWL has arrived at their weight reduction goal!

Pounds

In the UK it's normal to measure body weight. By way of instance, an individual gauging 250 pounds could get the aim of shedding 100 pounds to arrive at a goal weight 150 lbs. When estimating weight loss using BMI dimensions it is crucial to compare weight and weight reduction goals and body tallness. Therefore, Excessive Body Weight (EBW) and Excessive Weight reduction (EWL) are often used.

Overabundance Body Weight

EBW is the amount of bodyweight you've got in an overabundance of your goal weight. The normal BMI go is approximately 24. The ideal body weight for a single of tallness of 5 ft 7 inches is approximately 150 lbs. On the off probability that you weigh 250 lbs, at the point we calculate your EBW to become 100 lbs.

Overabundance weight reduction

EWL is the degree of your EBW which you shed. We guess EWL by dividing the number of pounds lost by the number of pounds on your EBW. As an example, if your own EBW is 100 lbs and you lose 45 pounds, your EWL is 45 percent.

Give me the opportunity to quantify that statement. If the scale is tumbling at a rotational motion, giving you continuous and fantastic misfortunes for quite some time, constantly, and without hindrance; at that point, the scale probably is not the Debbie for you.

And then there are all the people.

Verified actuality. I claim a scale. There was a point in time I once believed that decision would guarantee my programmed inversion back into the 327 pounds; the person I had been the afternoon of my health care procedure. Inquisitively, here I am, nearly 8 years post-operation, holding and lasting with 120 pounds. weight reduction.

Go figure.

In any instance, I am not here to convince you to concede the scale. This might give rise to a revolt and frankly, I do not have a home safety frame. Instead, I want you to look at some unique dimensions to keep tabs on your own development instead of simply looking at the scale.

What is the % extra bodyweight loss?

One step you ought to consider is the percentage of wealth body fat loss. That's really what it feels like. It is the level of this amount of weight that you want to shed, that you've just lost. (Do these words seem tangled for you as they do to me?)

In the Bariatric Foodie Facebook and Twitter accounts, we now intermittently assess our percent EBW (as I call it for short). Every time I get it done, folks get so optimistic. This amount enables you to feel path superior to the scale as it indicates that you're so close to where you want to be. It disposes of that"150 pounds Is exceptionally thin... or if I opt for 130?" business. It disposes of those X, Y and Y dropped 7,085 pounds. Their first two weeks following medical operation and I am at a slowdown" business. It centers around you in about you and your progress and provides you just how far you've come.

Prepared to work out how to get it done? It is mad basic!
One approach to figure your % extra bodyweight missing

(Compulsory Disclaimer: I'm conferring the way to do so, figuring in the way it had been taught to me. It's probably your bariatric careful clinic as of today's figures; this for you is determined by somewhat extraordinary math. On the off probability, they do always, always, always go with what your attentive practice says more than what I say. I am not a curative pro and do not play on t.v.!)

1. Take your start weight and subtract your goal weight. (I could not care less what amount you use to describe those... your own body, your choice!) As an example, if your start weight is 300 pounds. Additionally, your goal weight is 150, 300 - 150 = 150. This is the thing which you use as your prosperity body weight.

2. Next, visit this speed adding machine and look into the following column. (_____ is what amount of _____?) at the primary box place just how much weight you've lost up to now in pounds. (Or kg or anything you use... just attempt to use that

equal measure in the following box.) From the following box place the step of your prosperity body fat (that the aftereffect of #1).

3. Press "determine" The outcome is the % EBW.

What I enjoy about this estimation is that it provides that you're so close to where you want to be. From the preceding model, assume that person (whose EBW = 150) has lost 82 pounds. That suggests they've dropped 54.6percent of the prosperity body weight. That suggests that a person is more than most of the way to wherever they're trying to be.

This likewise suggests the individual is remarkable.
Use This Advice for Good, Not Evil!

At the stage, once we have a gander at the number on the scale, sometimes we get frustrated by that which we figure we ought to view, or confounded about the grounds which we simply don't have the foggiest notion what "average" is, especially on ourselves. Estimating your own% of wealth bodyweight loss induces you to center around your progress minus the untidiness of the confounded background together with the scale.

A

In any scenario, be careful. Likewise, like I do not want anyone getting too hung up about the scale, then you shouldn't get overly hung up with this amount. It is one of many measurements you along with your bariatric team can utilize to display your progress and just like using the scale, it is really the layout that matters. So, use this information carefully!

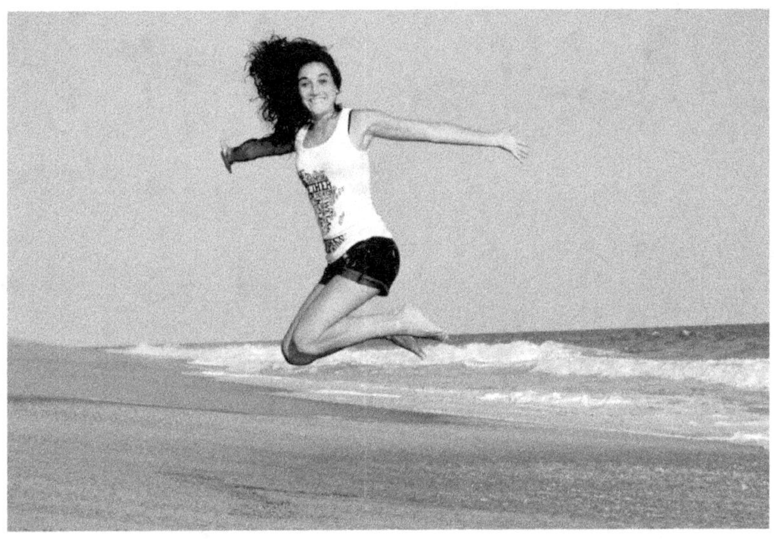

CHAPTER FIVE
20 RECIPES

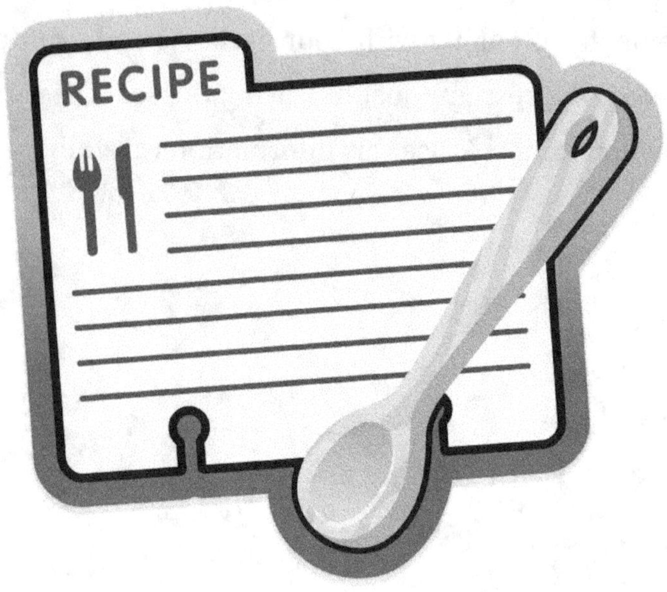

1) Crunchy banana yogurt

Banana and yogurt area ideal low-carb breakfast mix that will keep you going until lunchtime. The banana adds sweetness with no necessity for additional sugar, which along with the seeds bring a pleasing crunch. As a portion of an Irregular diet program, 1 serving provides Your everyday slice of two of your 3 daily low carb dairy pieces fruit; this meal supplies 149 mph portion.

Ingredients

340g/12oz fat-free organic Greek-style yogurt

1 banana, peeled and chopped

15g/1/2ounce mixed seeds (pumpkin, sesame, and sunflower) (or utilize toasted flaked almonds)

Technique

1. Split the yogurt between 2 little bowls. Scatter the banana on top.

2. Sprinkle with nuts or seeds and function.

Recipe Tips

Be aware of mixed bags of pumpkin, sesame, and sunflower seeds and watch your portion size carefully as they're extremely high in calories.

2) *Jumbo prawns with garlic and tomatoes*

This fiery dish of prawns, garlic, and tomatoes is ideal to warm you on a chilly winter night. If you would like to turn the heat down usage of less chili or not in any way. As a portion of an irregular diet program, 1 serving supplies 2 of the 6 daily vegetable parts. This meal supplies 180 mph portion.

Ingredients

1 tablespoon moderate olive oil

2 garlic tsp, very thinly sliced

1 red chili, deseeded and finely chopped (or use 1/2 tsp dried chili tsp)

150g/51/2ounce cherry tomatoes halved

1/2 lemon, the juice just

250g/9oz jumbo king prawns, cooked, peeled and deveined

3 heaped tbsp roughly chopped flat-leaf parsley

floor black pepper

160g/6oz green beans, steamed, to function

Technique

1. Heat the oil in a tiny skillet on low heat. Add the garlic and chili and cook very gently for 5 minutes until the garlic is quite soft but not colored, stirring periodically.

2. Add the berries and lemon juice and cook for 2 minutes or until starting to soften. Stir in the prawns and cook for 2-3 minutes, stirring until the berries are well softened and the prawns are warm through.

3. Remove the pan from the heat, stir in the parsley, season with a great deal of pepper and serve with the beans.

3) *Poached eggs with tomatoes and bacon*

A great alternative to the conventional fry-up that is low in calories but full of flavor. Poached eggs are an excellent way to generate breakfast somewhat lighter and amazingly simple to cook. As a portion of an Irregular diet program, 1 serving provides Your daily salty meals, 1 of the 6 daily vegetable parts. This meal supplies 212 mph portion.

Ingredients

2 large peeled berries, halved

4 rashers smoked back bacon; all visible fat removed

Two medium free-range eggs

floor black pepper

Technique

1. Preheat the grill to the hottest setting. Set the berries on a rack above a grill pan lined with foil. Season with pepper.

2. Grill for 3 minutes, then add the bacon and grill for a further 4 minutes, then turning the bacon after two minutes so it is lightly browned on each side.

3. Meanwhile, half-fill a medium pan with water and then bring it to the boil. Crack the eggs into two bowls. Turn down the heat so the water is bubbling quite softly. Gradually add the eggs into the water and then cook for 3 minutes until the white is set; however, the yolk stays runny.

4. With a slotted spoon, then scoop the eggs from the water and split between 2 plates. Add the cooked tomatoes and bacon. Season with a little salt and pepper and serve.

4) *Italian style meatballs with courgette 'tagliatelle'*

This flavourful dish of Italian meatballs includes a wholesome twist by employing courgette ribbons rather than pasta -- a simple way to cut calories. As a portion of an Irregular diet program, 1 serving supplies 3 of the 6 daily vegetable parts. This meal supplies a 219 mph portion.

Ingredients

For the meatballs

    250g/9oz extra lean beef mince (5 percent fat or less)
    1 little onion, very finely chopped
    1 teaspoon dried mixed herbs

calorie controlled cooking petroleum spray

1 garlic tsp, crushed

227g/8oz may chopped berries

2 tablespoons finely shredded fresh basil leaves, plus extra to garnish

For your courgette 'tagliatelle'

Two moderate courgettes, trimmed and deseeded

sea salt and freshly ground black pepper

Technique

1. Put the beef, half of the onion, half of the combined herbs, and a pinch of pepper and salt in a bowl and combine well. Divide into 10 small balls.

2. Spray a moderate non-stick skillet with a little oil and cook the meatballs for 5-7 minutes, turning occasionally until browned on all sides. Transfer to a plate.

3. For the sauce, then place the skillet in precisely the exact same pan and cook on a very low heat for 3 minutes, stirring. Add the garlic and cook for a couple of seconds.

4. Stir in the berries, 300ml/10fl oz water, the rest blended herbs, and shredded basil. Bring to the boil, stirring. Return the meatballs to the pan, then reduce the heat to a simmer and cook for 20 minutes, stirring occasionally until the sauce is thick and the meatballs are cooked throughout.

5. Meanwhile, half-fill a medium pan with water and bring to the boil. Use a vegetable peeler to pare off the courgettes to ribbons. Cook the courgette from the boiling water for a minute then drain.

6. Split the courgette ribbons between 2 plates and top with the meatballs and sauce. Garnish with basil leaves.
Recipe Tips

You can prepare the meal the night before, then reheat in the microwave if you prefer.

5) *Vegetable and wheat Balti*

Attempt this vegetable and chicken Balti to get a wholesome curry that's fast and simple to prepare. As a portion of an Irregular diet program, 1 serving provides 1 of your 3-daily low-carb dairy parts, two of your 6 daily vegetable parts. This meal supplies 341 kcal, 40g protein, 30.5g carbohydrate (of which

20.5grams sugars), 6g fat (of which 1.5g saturates), 9g fiber and 0.6g salt per portion.

Ingredients

calorie controlled cooking oil spray

1 moderate onion, thinly sliced

4 chicken thighs, boned and skinned

1 reddish pepper, deseeded and cut to 3cm/1in balls

1 yellowish tsp, deseeded and cut into 3cm/1in balls

1 tablespoon cornflour

150g/51/2ounce fat-free All-natural yogurt

1 tablespoon medium or moderate curry powder

Two garlic cloves, thinly chopped

227g/8oz tin chopped berries

3 tablespoons finely chopped fresh coriander, plus extra to garnish

freshly ground black pepper

Technique

1. Spray a large, deep, non-stick skillet or wok with oil and set over medium heat. Add the onion and cook for five minutes, stirring frequently until well softened and lightly browned.

2. Meanwhile, trim each of the visible fat off the chicken thighs, cut each one into four pieces and season with black pepper.

3. Add the broccoli and chicken to the pan with the onion and cook for 3 minutes, turning occasionally.

4. In a small bowl, mix the cornflour with 2 tbsp cold water and then stir into the yogurt until completely blended.

5. Sprinkle the curry powder on the lettuce and chicken, add the garlic and cook for 30 minutes.

6. Hint the berries into the pan, then add the yogurt mix, 150ml/31/2fl ounces of water and coriander.

7. Bring to a gentle simmer and cook for 20-25 minutes, stirring occasionally till the chicken is tender and the sauce is thick. Season with freshly ground black pepper to taste and garnish with coriander.

6) *Lamb and flageolet bean stew*

This is a heating stew ideal for filling one up on a chilly day. Do not be put off by the lengthy cooking period, this can be a simple one-pot dinner which can benefit you for your patience. As a portion of an irregular diet program, 1 serving provides - your daily salty meals - 3 of your 6 daily vegetable parts. This meal supplies a 288 mph portion.

Ingredients

1 teaspoon olive oil

350g/12oz lean lamb, cubed

16 pickling onions

1 garlic clove, crushed

600ml/20fl ounce lamb stock (created with concentrated liquid inventory)

200g could chopped berries

1 bouquet garni

2 x 400g cans flageolet beans, emptied and rinsed

320g/11oz green beans

250g/9oz cherry tomatoes

freshly ground black pepper

Technique

1. Heat the oil in a flameproof casserole or saucepan, add the lamb and simmer for 3-4 minutes until browned. Remove the lamb from the casserole and set aside.

2. Add the garlic and onions into the pan and simmer for 4-5 minutes, or until the onions are starting to brown.

3. Pour the carrot and any juices to the pan. Add the stock, tomatoes, bouquet garni and legumes. Bring to the boil, stirring,

then cover and simmer for 1 hour or until the lamb is only tender.

4. Meanwhile, bring a bowl of water to the boil and blanch the green beans. Put in a bowl of ice-cold water.

5. Add the cherry tomatoes to the stew and season well with freshly ground black pepper. Continue to simmer for 10 minutes.

6. Split the stew between four plates, put the green beans together and function.
Recipe Tips

This dish can be made the night before and warmed up.
Hearty vegetable soup

This hearty vegetable soup is packed full of goodness and flavor, perfect to warm you on a chilly night. When eating on a limited day of an intermittent diet, replace the carrots using deseeded yellow peppers. Included in an Intermittent diet program, 1 serving provides Your daily salty meals with 3 of the 5 daily vegetable parts. This meal supplies a 219 mph portion.
Ingredients

calorie controlled cooking oil spray

1 moderate onion, sliced

Two garlic cloves, thinly sliced

Two celery sticks, trimmed and finely sliced

Two moderate carrots or two yellow peppers, cut to 2cm/1in balls

400g/14oz tin chopped berries

1 vegetable inventory block

1 teaspoon dried mixed herbs

400g/14oz tin butter beans, emptied and rinsed

1 mind youthful spring greens (roughly 125g/41/2ounce), trimmed and chopped

sea salt and freshly milled black pepper

Technique

1. Spray a big skillet with oil and then cook the garlic, onion, carrots and celery or peppers lightly for 10 minutes, stirring frequently until softened.

2. Insert 750ml/26fl ounce water and the chopped tomatoes. Crumble over the stock cube and stir in the dried herbs. Bring to the boil, then lower the heat to a simmer and cook for 20 minutes.

3. Season the soup with salt and pepper and then put in the spring greens and butterbeans. Return to a simmer and cook for

a further 3-4 minutes until the greens have been softened. Season to taste and serve in deep bowls.

Recipe Tips

Double the recipe if you fancy eating it over a few days.

The butter beans may be substituted for other legumes out of your store cupboard in case you don't have some.

7) *Berry yogurt*

A luscious, fruity yogurt which produces a satisfying breakfast. Using frozen berries saves money and they create a flavourful juice since they thaw. As a portion of an irregular diet program, 1 serving provides Your everyday slice of fruit, and two of your 3 daily low carb dairy pieces. This meal supplies a 149 mph portion.

Ingredients

175g/6oz frozen mixed berries, defrosted

340g/12oz fat-free Greek yogurt

10g/1/4ounce flaked almonds, toasted

Technique

1. Spoon the yogurt into two glasses, then top with half of the berries, then repeat the layers.

2. Sprinkle with the flaked almonds and serve.

Recipe Tips

You can toast the almonds in a dry skillet pan or purchase the ready toasted type.

8) *Garlic mushroom frittata*

Garlic and mushrooms bring amazing flavor for this super-low-calorie, easy-to-make frittata. Serve with salad for a very simple and delicious lunch. As a portion of an Intermittent diet program, 1 serving supplies 3 of the 6 daily vegetable parts. This meal supplies 243 kcal, 14g protein, 3.5g carbohydrate (of which 3g sugars), 14g fat (of which 4g saturates), 2.5g fiber and 0.6g salt per part.

Ingredients

low-carb spray
250g/9oz chestnut mushrooms, sliced
1 little garlic clove, crushed

1 tablespoon thinly sliced fresh chives

4 big free-range eggs, crushed

freshly ground black pepper

For your salad

1 Little gem lettuce, leaves split

100g/31/2ounce cherry tomatoes halved

1/3 cucumber, cut into balls

Technique

1. Spray a little, flame-proof skillet with oil and set on high heat. (The bottom of the pan should not be wider than roughly 18cm/7in.) Stir-fry the mushrooms in 3 batches for 2-3 minutes, or until softened and lightly browned. Hint the boiled mushrooms into a sieve over a bowl to catch any juices -- you do not need the mushrooms to become soggy.

2. Return all the mushrooms into the pan and stir in the garlic and chives, and a pinch of pepper. Cook for a further minute, then lower to reduce the heat.

3. Preheat the grill to the hottest setting. Pour the eggs over the mushrooms. Cook for five minutes, or until nearly set.

4. Set the pan under the grill for 3-4 minutes, or until set.

5. Combine the salad ingredients in a bowl.

6. Remove from the grill and then loosen the faces of the frittata with a round-bladed knife. Turn onto a board and cut into wedges. Serve warm or cold with all the salad.

Recipe Tips

Ensure you utilize a tiny non-invasive skillet, which means that your frittata is thick and nice.

Extra-lean salad and legumes.

Forget fat-packed takeaway hamburgers. Tuck into our homemade 'fakeaway' deal. As a portion of an irregular diet program, 1 serving supplies 2 of the 6 daily vegetable parts. This meal supplies 255 kcal, 36g protein, 6g carbohydrate (of which 5.5grams sugars), 7g fat (of which 2.5g saturates), 3g fiber and 0.4g salt per part.

Ingredients

low-carb spray

1/2 little onion, finely chopped

100g/31/2ounce Portobello mushrooms, finely chopped

250g/9oz extra-lean beef mince (under 5 percent fat)

2 teaspoons finely chopped fresh thyme (or 1/2 teaspoon dried thyme)

freshly ground black pepper

For your salad

1 Little Gem lettuce, leaves split

120g/41/2ounce cherry berries, sliced

1/3 cucumber, chopped

Technique

1. Spray a tiny skillet with oil and then cook the mushrooms and onion over a moderate heat for 5 minutes, or until nicely softened, stirring frequently. Hint into a heatproof bowl and leave to cool for 5 minutes.

2. Add the steak, thyme and a lot of ground black pepper. Mix well and shape into two chunks. Flatten into burger shapes, each round 2cm/3/4in thick.

3. Wash out the pan and then go back to the hob. Spray with a bit more oil and then cook the hamburgers over medium-low heat for 10 minutes, turning occasionally, until browned on the outside and cooked through indoors.

4. Serve the burgers with lettuce, tomatoes, and pineapple.

Recipe Tips

If you are not keen on beef, then try making with minced chicken or turkey breast instead.

9) *Cinnamon porridge with grated pear*

This porridge is made from the water and skimmed milk to keep the calories. Just small ground cinnamon makes it taste sweeter without including calories and it's topped with hot grated pear. As a portion of an Irregular diet program, 1 serving supplies a half part of your 6 daily vegetable parts, 1 of your milk pieces and 219 kcal.

Ingredients

60g/21/4ounce Tank porridge oats

1/4 tsp ground cinnamon, and a little to scatter

300ml/10fl oz semi-skimmed milk

1 ripe medium pear

1 leash lemon

Technique

1. Sct the ginger and cinnamon into a skillet with the milk and cook on a low-medium heat for 4-5 minutes, stirring continuously until creamy and rich. Pour into two heavy bowls.

2. Coarsely grate the pear and put on top of this porridge. Squeeze over the lemon juice and sprinkle with a very small pinch of ground cinnamon.

Recipe Tips

It is very important to use jumbo oats, instead of instant oats since they take more time to digest.

10) *Chermoula tofu and roasted veggies*

Tofu beautifully absorbs the flavors of chermoula within this dish. Serve with roasted vegetables for a hearty vegetarian meal. As a portion of an irregular diet program, 1 serving supplies 2 of the 6 daily vegetable parts. This meal supplies a 182 mph portion.

Ingredients

For your chermoula tofu

25g/1oz coriander, finely chopped

3 garlic tsp, sliced

1 teaspoon cumin seeds, lightly crushed

1 lemon, finely grated rind

1/2 teaspoon dried crushed chilies

1 tablespoon olive oil

250g/9oz tofu

For your roasted veggies

Two red onions, quartered

Two courgettes, thickly chopped

2 reddish peppers, deseeded and chopped

2 yellowish peppers, deseeded and chopped

1 little aubergine, thickly chopped

low-carb spray

pinch salt

Technique

1. Preheat the oven to 200ºC/180ºC Fan/ Gas 6.

2. For your chermoula, combine the garlic, coriander, cumin, lemon rind and chilies along with the oil and a bit of salt in a small bowl.

3. Pat the tofu dry on kitchen paper and then cut it in half. Cut each half into thin pieces. Distribute the chermoula liberally on the pieces.

4. Scatter the vegetables in a roasting tin and then spray oil. Bake for approximately 45 minutes, until lightly browned, turning the components a couple of times during cooking.

5. Arrange the tofu pieces over the veggies, together with the side spread together with all the chermoula uppermost, and bake for a further 10-15 minutes, or until the tofu is lightly colored.

6. Split the lettuce and kale between four plates and serve.

11)   *Hearty vegetable soup*

This hearty vegetable soup is packed full of goodness and flavor, perfect to warm you on a chilly night. When eating on a limited day of an intermittent diet, then replace the carrots using deseeded yellow peppers. Included in an Intermittent diet program, 1 serving provides Your daily salty meals 3 of the 5 daily vegetable parts. This meal supplies a 219 mph portion.

Ingredients

calorie controlled cooking oil spray

1 moderate onion, sliced

Two garlic cloves, thinly sliced

Two celery sticks, trimmed and finely sliced

Two moderate carrots or two yellow peppers, cut to 2cm/1in balls

400g/14oz tin chopped berries

1 vegetable inventory block

1 teaspoon dried mixed herbs

400g/14oz tin butter beans, emptied and rinsed

1 mind youthful spring greens (roughly 125g/41/2ounce), trimmed and chopped

sea salt and freshly milled black pepper

Technique

1. Spray a big skillet with oil and then cook the garlic, onion, carrots and celery or peppers lightly for 10 minutes, stirring frequently until softened.

2. Insert 750ml/26fl ounce water and the chopped tomatoes. Crumble over the stock cube and stir in the dried herbs. Bring to boil, then lower the heat to a simmer and cook for 20 minutes.

3. Season the soup with salt and pepper and then put in the spring greens and butterbeans. Return to a simmer and cook for a further 3-4 minutes until the greens have been softened. Season to taste and serve in deep bowls.

Recipe Tips

Double the recipe if you fancy eating it over a few days.

The butter beans may be substituted for other legumes out of your store cupboard in case you don't have some.

12)   ***Peppered beef with salad leaves***

This is a quick supper, ideal for a busy day. Horseradish sauce adds a kick into the salad dressing table. As a portion of an Irregular diet program, 1 serving supplies 1 of the 6 daily vegetable parts and 148 kcal. If eating it within a daily Intermittent diet, also enjoy a bit of fruit on this meal (approximately 70 calories).

Ingredients

two thick-cut sirloin steaks, about 175g/6oz incomplete, fat trimmed

1 teaspoon colored peppercorns, coarsely crushed

rough salt tsp

60g/21/4ounce natural yogurt

1/2 tsp horseradish sauce (to taste)

1/2 garlic clove, crushed

50g/2oz mixed green salad leaves

30g/11/4ounce button mushrooms, chopped

1/2 red onion, thinly chopped

1 teaspoon olive oil

salt and freshly milled black pepper

Technique

1. Rub the steaks with the crushed peppercorns and salt flakes.

2. Mix together the yogurt, horseradish sauce and garlic and season to taste with salt and freshly ground black pepper. Insert the salad leaves, mushrooms and most of the red onion and toss lightly.

3. Heat the oil in a skillet, add the steaks and cook on high heat for two minutes, or until browned. Turn over and cook for a further two minutes for medium-rare, 3-4 minutes for medium or 5 minutes for well done. Put the beef onto a hot plate and let it rest for a couple of minutes.

4. Spoon the salad leaves to the center of two serving dishes. Thinly slice the beans and arrange the pieces on top. Garnish with the remaining red onion.

13)   <u>*Caponata ratatouille*</u>

Ratatouille is a wonderfully warming vegetable noodle originating from Provence. Fantastic for satisfying vegetarians and meat-eaters alike. As a portion of an Irregular diet program, 1 serving provides Your daily salty meals 2 of the 6 daily vegetable parts This meal supplies 90 mph portion.

Ingredients

1 tablespoon olive oil

750g/1lb 10oz aubergines, cut into 1cm/11/2in balls

1 big onion, cut into 1cm/11/2in balls

3 celery sticks, roughly sliced

2 big beef berries, peeled and deseeded

1 teaspoon sliced thyme

1/4-1/2 tsp cayenne pepper

2 tablespoon capers, emptied

little handful pitted green tsp

4 tablespoons white wine vinegar

1 tablespoon sugar

1-2 tablespoon cocoa powder (discretionary)

freshly ground black pepper

To garnish

chopped tsp, toasted

chopped tsp

Technique

1. Heat the oil in a non-stick skillet till quite hot, add the aubergine and simmer for approximately 15 minutes, or until quite soft. Add a little boiling water to prevent sticking if needed.

2. Meanwhile, put the celery and onion in a large saucepan with a little water. Cook for 5 minutes, or until tender but still firm.

3. Add the berries, coriander, cayenne pepper and aubergine to the saucepan. Cook for 15 minutes, stirring periodically. Add the capers, olives, vinegar, sugar and cocoa powder and cook for 2-3 minutes.

1. Season with freshly ground black pepper. Split between 6 bowls, garnish with the toasted almonds and parsley and serve.
Recipe Tips

If you do not fancy aubergines, you may use courgettes. Simply add the courgettes in precisely the exact same time as the berries.

14)   Healthy scrambled eggs

Scrambled eggs have been made extra special by including smoked salmon. Serve with fresh watercress and broiled vine tomatoes to get a more satisfying breakfast. As a portion of an Irregular diet strategy, 1 serving supplies your daily salty meals. Each serving supplies 263kcal, 21g protein, 10g carbs (of which 10g sugars), 14g fat (of which 3.5g saturates), 4g fiber and 1g salt.

Ingredients

8 midi vine berries, halved

low-carb spray

3 big free-range eggs

35g/11/4ounce smoked salmon, roughly sliced

1 tablespoon sliced chives

25g/1oz new watercress, to function

freshly ground black pepper

Technique

1. Season the berries. Heat a pan sprayed with cooking spray oil over medium heat, add the tomatoes and cook for 2-3 minutes, until softened, stirring from time to time but not dividing the berries.

2. Meanwhile, beat the eggs in a bowl with a few peppers. Stir in the salmon and chives and pour into a saucepan.

3. Cook very gently for 3-4 minutes, stirring gradually, until the eggs are lightly bubbling. Remove from the heat and simmer for a Couple of Seconds.

4. Divide the berries between 2 plates and serve together with all the scrambled eggs along with the watercress.

15)   ***Red mullet with chopped tomatoes***

Baking fish is a simple way to reduce calories without compromising flavor. Serve alongside baked tomatoes to get a nutritious evening meal. As a portion of an Irregular diet program, 1 serving supplies 2 of the 6 daily vegetable parts and 248 kcal.

Ingredients

for Those berries

    375g/13oz mixed yellow and red cherry tomatoes

    320g/111/2ounce fine green beans, trimmed

    Two garlic cloves, finely chopped

    2 tablespoon lemon juice

    low-carb spray

    salt and freshly milled black pepper

For your red mullet

8 red mullet fillets, roughly 100g/ 3 1/2ounce each
1 lemon, finely grated rind just
2 tsp infant capers, emptied
Two spring onions, finely chopped

To garnish

2 tbsp sliced tsp
8 caperberries

Technique

1. Preheat the oven to 200ºC/180ºC Fan/Gas 6.

2. Set the tomatoes in an ovenproof dish with all the garlic, beans, lemon juice and then juice together with the oil. Season with salt and freshly ground black pepper and blend well. Bake for 10 minutes, or until the berries and beans are tender.

3. Meanwhile, tear off 4 large sheets of foil and line with non-stick paper. Put two fish fillets on each piece of paper, then scatter over the lemon rind, capers, and spring onions, season with salt and freshly ground black pepper. Fold on the paper-

lined transparency and scrunch the edges together to seal. Put the parcels on a large skillet.

4. Set the fish parcels near the veggies in the oven and bake for a further 8-10 minutes, or until the flesh flakes easily when pressed in the middle with a knife.

5. Spoon the vegetables on to four serving dishes and top each with 2 bass fillets. Garnish with the parsley and caperberries and function.

16)   *Vegetables with red pepper rouille*

Roasted vegetables don't have to be dull; flavor with saffron and function with a smoky red pepper rouille to make a yummy vegetarian dinner. With this recipe, you'll require a liquidizer or food processor. Included in an Intermittent diet program, 1 serving supplies 2 of the 6 daily vegetable parts. This meal supplies a 142 mph portion.

Ingredients

4 tablespoons olive oil

2-3 garlic cloves, finely chopped

3 big pinches of saffron ribbons

3 blended orange and red peppers, cored, deseeded and each cut into 6 bits

3 courgettes, roughly 100g/31/2ounce each, chopped into 2.5cm/1in balls

Two onions, cut into wedges

salt and freshly milled black pepper

For the rouille

4 plum berries, about 250g/9oz in Complete

1 reddish tsp, cored, deseeded and quartered

1 garlic clove, finely chopped

large pinch of earth smoked paprika

1 tablespoon olive oil

Technique

1. Preheat the oven to 220°C/200°C Fan/Gas 7.

2. Set the oil for those veggies in a big plastic bag with garlic, saffron and some pepper and salt. Add the veggies, hold the top border of the bag to seal and throw together. Put aside for at least 30 minutes.

3. Meanwhile for your rouille, set the pepper and tomatoes in a small roasting tin. Sprinkle with garlic, smoked paprika, some

pepper, and salt. Then drizzle the boil and simmer for 15 minutes. Allow cooling.

4. Peel the skins from the tomatoes and pepper. Purée the flesh at a liquidizer or food processor with any juices in the roasting tin till smooth. Spoon into a serving bowl and put aside, keep warm.

5. Hint the saffron vegetables to a large roasting tin and cook in the oven for 15-20 minutes, turning once, until browned.

6. Spoon the vegetables on to individual dishes and serve with spoonsful of this rouille.

17) ***Stir-fried pork with soy and ginger sauce***

This low-carb, stir-fried pork is fast and simple while still providing flavor and assisting you in your way to becoming five a day. As a portion of an Irregular diet program, 1 serving provides Your daily salty meals 3 of your 5 daily vegetable parts. This meal supplies 250 mph portion.

Ingredients

250g/9oz pork tenderloin, all visible fat removed, cut into balls

1 teaspoon cornflour

2 tbsp dark soy sauce

low-carb spray

150g/51/2ounce button mushrooms, chopped

2 reddish peppers, deseeded and chopped

75g/21/2ounce mangetout, trimmed

15g/1/2ounce fresh root ginger, cut into thin matchsticks

1 garlic clove, thinly chopped

4 spring onions, cut into short lengths

freshly ground black pepper

Technique

1. Season the pork with pepper. Mix the cornflour with 2 tbsp of cold water till smooth, then stir in the soy sauce.

2. Spray a large skillet, or heavy skillet, with cooking spray and set over high heat. Stir-fry the pork for 1-2 minutes, or until lightly browned but not cooked through. Transfer to a plate.

3. Return the pan to the heat, reduce the heat a bit and spray more oil. Stir-fry the pepper and mushrooms for 2 minutes. Add the mangetout and cook for a moment. Add the garlic, ginger and spring onions and simmer for a couple of seconds.

4. Return the pork to the pan and then pour the soy sauce mix. Cook for 1-2 minutes, or until the sauce has thickened and the pork is cooked through. Drink immediately.

Moroccan baked eggs

Baked eggs would be the ideal dish for an idle brunch. Should you prefer your eggs hot just put in a little chili powder. As a portion of an Intermittent diet program, 1 serving supplies 2 of the 6 daily vegetable parts. This meal supplies 170 mph portion. If eaten within a daily Intermittent diet, additionally enjoy 200ml skimmed milk (70 calories).

Ingredients

1/2 tablespoon olive oil

1/2 onion, chopped

1 garlic tsp, chopped

1/2 tsp ras el hanout

pinch floor cinnamon

1/2 tsp ground coriander

400g/14oz cherry tomatoes, chopped

2 tbsp sliced coriander

2 tablespoons eggs

salt and freshly milled black pepper

Technique

1. Prcheat the oven to 220°C/200°C Fan/Gas 7.

2. Heat the oil in a skillet, add the garlic and onion and cook for 6-7 minutes, or until tender. Stir in the spices and cook, stirring, for a further minute.

3. Add the tomatoes and season well with pepper and salt, then simmer gently for 8-10 minutes.

4. Scatter over 1 tbsp of coriander, then split the tomato mix between two individual ovenproof dishes. Break an egg into each dish.

5. Bake for 8-10 minutes until the egg whites are set but the yolks are still slightly runny. Cook for a further 2-3 minutes if you want the eggs to be cooked through.

6. Scatter over the remaining coriander and function.
Recipe Tips

This dish would also make a fantastic fast dinner if functioned along with a leafy green salad.

18)   _Chilli and coriander fish parcel_

Baking fish is an excellent way to reduce calories. Give the fish additional oomph with chili and coriander. With this recipe, you'll need a blender or a food processor. Included in an Intermittent diet program, 1 serving supplies 1 of the 6 daily vegetable parts and 148 calories.

Ingredients

125g/41/2ounce cod, coley or haddock fillet

2 tsp lemon juice

1 tablespoon fresh coriander leaves

1 garlic clove, roughly chopped

1 green chili, deseeded and sliced

1/4 tsp sugar

2 tsp organic yogurt

80g/3oz mangetout, steamed, to function

Technique

1. Preheat the oven to 200ºC/180ºC Fan/Gas 6.

2. Put the fish in a non-metallic dish and sprinkle with the lemon juice. Cover and leave in the refrigerator to simmer for 15-20 minutes.

3. Set the garlic, coriander, and chili into a food processor or blender and process until the mixture forms a paste. Add the sugar yogurt and temporarily proceed to blend.

4. Place the fish on a sheet of transparency. Coat the fish on both sides using all the glue. Collect the foil loosely and twist over in the top to seal. Return to the refrigerator for 1 hour.

5. Set the package onto a baking tray and bake for approximately 15 minutes, or till the fish is just cooked. Serve with all the mangetout.

19)   *Red mullet with chopped tomatoes*

Baking fish is a simple way to reduce calories without compromising flavor. Serve alongside baked tomatoes to get a nutritious evening meal. As a portion of an Irregular diet program, 1 serving supplies 2 of the 6 daily vegetable parts and 248 kcal.

Ingredients

for Those berries

375g/13oz mixed yellow and red cherry tomatoes
320g/111/2ounce fine green beans, trimmed
Two garlic cloves, finely chopped

2 tablespoon lemon juice

low-carb spray

salt and freshly milled black pepper

For your red mullet

8 red mullet fillets, roughly 100g/31/2ounce each

1 lemon, finely grated rind just

2 tsp infant capers, emptied

Two spring onions, finely chopped

To garnish

2 tbsp sliced tsp

8 caperberries

Technique

1. Preheat the oven to 200ºC/180ºC Fan/Gas 6.

2. Set the tomatoes in an ovenproof dish with all the garlic, beans, lemon juice and then juice together with the oil. Season with salt and freshly ground black pepper and blend well. Bake for 10 minutes, or until the berries and beans are tender.

3. Meanwhile, tear off 4 large sheets of foil and line with non-stick paper. Put two fish fillets on each piece of paper, then scatter over the lemon rind, capers, and spring onions; season with salt and freshly ground black pepper. Fold on the paper-lined transparency and scrunch the edges together to seal. Put the parcels on a large skillet.

4. Set the fish parcels near the veggies in the oven and bake for a further 8-10 minutes, or until the flesh flakes easily when pressed in the middle with a knife.

5. Spoon the vegetables on to four serving dishes and top each with 2 bass fillets. Garnish with the parsley and caperberries and function.

20)   *Peppered beef with salad leaves*

This is a quick supper, ideal for a busy day. Horseradish sauce adds a kick into the salad dressing table. As a portion of an Irregular diet program, 1 serving supplies 1 of the 6 daily vegetable parts and 148 kcal. If eaten within a daily Intermittent diet, also enjoy a bit of fruit on this meal (approximately 70 calories).

Ingredients

two thick-cut sirloin steaks, about 175g/6oz incomplete, fat trimmed

1 teaspoon colored peppercorns, coarsely crushed

rough salt tsp

60g/21/4ounce natural yogurt

1/2 tsp horseradish sauce (to taste)

1/2 garlic clove, crushed

50g/2oz mixed green salad leaves

30g/11/4ounce button mushrooms, chopped

1/2 red onion, thinly chopped

1 teaspoon olive oil

salt and freshly milled black pepper

Technique

1. Rub the steaks with the crushed peppercorns and salt flakes.

2. Mix together the yogurt, horseradish sauce and garlic and season to taste with salt and freshly ground black pepper. Insert the salad leaves, mushrooms and most of the red onion and toss lightly.

3. Heat the oil in a skillet, add the steaks and cook on high heat for two minutes, or until browned. Turn over and cook for a further two minutes for medium-rare, 3-4 minutes for medium

or 5 minutes for well done. Put the beef onto a hot plate and let it rest for a couple of minutes.

4. Spoon the salad leaves to the center of two serving dishes. Thinly slice the beans and arrange the pieces on top. Garnish with the remaining red onion.

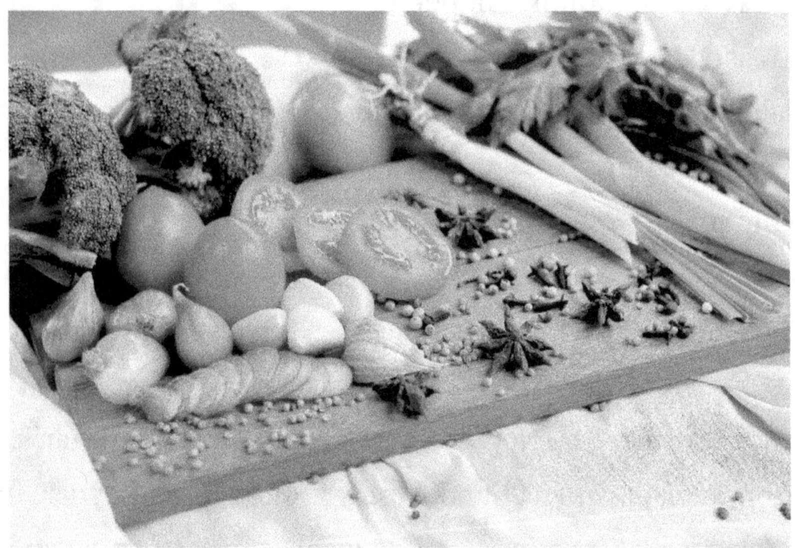

CHAPTER SIX
AUTOPHAGY AND ITS BENEFITS

Autophagy is your body's way of cleaning out cells that are damaged so that you can regenerate newer, healthy cells; this is according to Priya Khorana, Ph.D. in Nutrition Education from Columbia University.

"Automobile" is self-explanatory, and "phage" signifies consume. Therefore, the literal meaning of autophagy is "self-eating."

Additionally, it is known as "self-devouring." While this may seem like something you don't even need to happen for your body, it is helpful to your general wellness.

This is only because autophagy is an evolutionary self-preservation mechanism of the body that can get rid of the dysfunctional tissues and recycle elements of these toward mobile cleaning and repair, according to a board-certified cardiologist.

Petre clarifies that the goal of autophagy is to eliminate debris and self-regulate back to optimum smooth functioning.

"It is cleaning and recycling at the exact same time; like hitting a reset button to your entire body. Additionally, it boosts survival and adaptation as a response to different stressors and toxins accumulated within our own cells," she adds.

Which are the advantages of autophagy?

The main advantages of autophagy appear to come from the kind of anti-aging principles. Petre says it is best known as the body's method of turning back the clock and producing younger cells.

Khorana points out that when our cells are worried, autophagy is raised to be able to protect us, which can help improve our life span.

In addition, registered dietitian, Scott Keatley, RD, CDN, states that in times of starvation, autophagy keeps your system moving by breaking down cellular material and reusing it to get essential procedures.

"Obviously, that takes energy and cannot continue indefinitely, but it provides us more time to find nutrition," he adds.

At the cellular level, Petre states the advantages of autophagy as comprising:

Eliminating toxic proteins in the cells which are credited to neurodegenerative diseases, for example, Parkinson's and Alzheimer's disease

recycling remaining proteins

supplying energy and building blocks for cells which may still benefit from the fix

to a bigger scale, it arouses regeneration and wholesome cells

Autophagy is getting a great deal of focus for the role it could play in preventing or treating cancer also.

While all cancers begin from home kind of faulty cells, Petre states that the body needs to recognize and eliminate those cells frequently with autophagic processes. That is why some researchers are looking at the possibility that autophagy can diminish the chance of cancer.

Researchers consider that new studies will lead to insight to assist them in the goal of autophagy as a treatment for cancer.

Diet changes that may boost autophagy

Bear in mind that autophagy literally signifies "self-eating." So, it makes sense that intermittent fasting and ketogenic diets are proven to activate autophagy.

"Ketosis, a diet high in fat and reduced in carbohydrates brings the very same advantages of fasting, like a shortcut to cause exactly the identical favorable metabolic changes," she adds. "By not overpowering the body in having an external loading, it provides the body a rest to concentrate on its health and fix it."

From the keto diet, you receive about 75 percent of your daily calories from fat, and 5 to 10 percent of your calories from carbohydrates.

This change in calorie sources causes the human body to change its metabolic pathways. It will start to utilize fat for fuel rather than the sugar that is derived from carbs.

In reaction to this limitation, your body will start to begin to generate ketone bodies which have many protective results. Khorana says studies indicate that ketosis may also bring about starvation-induced autophagy, which has neuroprotective functions.

"Low sugar levels occur in the two diets and are connected to reduced insulin and high glucagon levels," explains Petre. And glucagon level is what initiates autophagy.

"If your system is low on sugar or ketosis, it attracts the positive pressure that wakes up the survival fixing mode," she adds.

One non-diet area that can play a role in causing autophagy is exercise. According to single creature research, bodily exercise can induce autophagy in organs which are a part of metabolic regulation procedures.

This may include the muscles, pancreas, liver, and adrenal tissue.
The most important thing is that

Autophagy will continue to get attention as investigators run more studies on the effect it has on our health.

For today, nutritional and health specialists like Khorana attest to the truth that there is still much we will need to know about autophagy, and the way to best promote it.

But if you are interested in attempting to excite autophagy on the human body, she recommends beginning by incorporating fasting and regular exercise in your routine.

But you must consult your physician if you are taking any drugs, pregnant, or want to get pregnant, or have a chronic condition, such as heart disease or diabetes.

Khorana warns that you are not invited quickly if you fall into any of the above-mentioned classes.

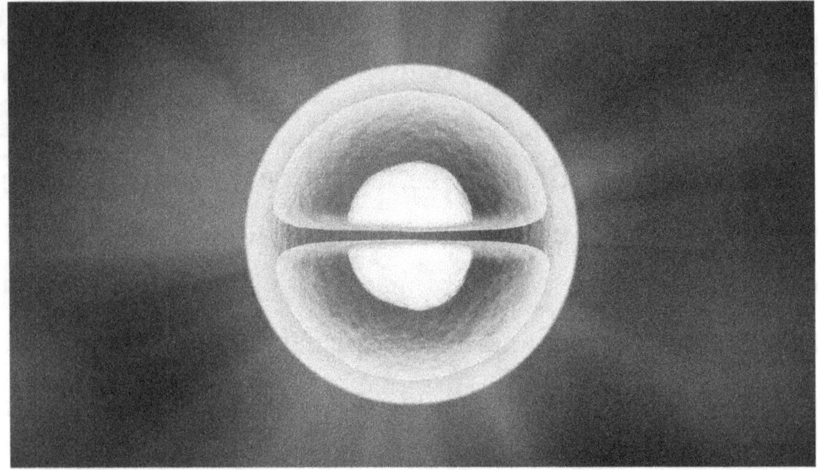

CHAPTER SEVEN
FOOD THAT BOOST AUTOPHAGY PROCESS

It is difficult to figure out the amount of exercise needed to change on the autophagy boost.

1. Water

Though you are not eating, it is important to remain hydrated for a lot of reasons, such as the wellbeing of essentially every significant organ in your system. The quantity of water which anyone individual must drink fluctuates, but you would like your pee for a light yellowish color at any time. Dark yellow urine indicates dehydration, which may lead to headaches, fatigue, and light-headedness. Couple that with restricted food, and it might be a recipe for disaster. If the idea of plain water does not provoke you, add a squeeze of lemon juice, a couple of mint leaves, or lemon pieces to your own water. It will be our little secret.

2. Avocado

It might appear counterintuitive to consume the highest calorie while trying to shed weight; however, the monounsaturated fat in avocado is extremely satiating. Research even discovered that adding a half of an avocado into your lunch can keep you full for hours.

3. Fish

There is a reason the Dietary guidelines suggest the ingestion of at least eight ounces of fish each week. Not only is it rich in healthful fats and protein, but it also contains considerable quantities of vitamin D. And if you are just eating a limited quantity of food through the day, do not need one, which produces additional nutrient-bang for your dollar? And of course, that restricting your calorie consumption might mess with your cognition fish is frequently considered a "brainfoods."

4. Cruciferous Veggies

Foods like broccoli, Brussels sprouts, and cauliflower are full of the f-word--fiber. When you are eating erratically, it is vital to eat fiber-rich foods which will keep you regular and protect against constipation. Fiber has the capacity to cause you to feel complete, which is something that you may want in case you cannot eat for 16 hours. Woof.

5. Potatoes

Repeat after me; not many white foods are poor. Case in point: Research has discovered potatoes to be among the most satiating foods. Another research discovered that eating berries as part of a healthy diet might aid with weight reduction. Sorry, French fries and potato chips do not count.

5. Beans and Legumes

Your favorite addition to chili might be your very best buddy on the IF lifestyle. Food, especially carbohydrates, provides energy for action. While we are not telling you how to carbo-load, it certainly would not hurt to throw a few low-carb carbohydrates, such as legumes and beans, in your eating program. Additionally, foods such as chickpeas, black beans, peas, and lentils are demonstrated to reduce body fat, even with no calorie restriction.

6. Probiotics

Do you understand exactly what the little critters on your gut are? Consistency and diversity. That means that they are not happy when they are hungry. When your gut is not happy, you might encounter some bothersome side effects, such as constipation. To counteract this unpleasantness, include probiotic-rich foods, such as kefir, kombucha or kraut, to a daily diet. The Farmhouse Culture Gut Shots are ideal for any 500-calorie daily because every 1.5-ounce shot is teeming with live probiotics (10 billion CFUs) for only 10 calories.

7. Berries

Your favorite smoothie improvement is ripe with essential nutrients. Strawberries are an excellent source of immune-boosting vitamin C, using over 100% of the daily value in 1 cup. And that is not the best part-- current research found that individuals who have a diet full of flavonoids, such as those in tomatoes and blueberries, had smaller gains in BMI on a 14-year interval than people who didn't eat berries.

8. Eggs

1 big egg contains six grams of protein plus cooks in minutes. Obtaining as much protein as you can is important for maintaining fullness and building muscle. One research discovered that men who ate an egg instead of a bagel were hungry and ate less during the day. To put it differently, once you're searching for something to do throughout your fasting interval, why not hard-boil some eggs?

9. Nuts

They are higher in calories than several other snacks, but nuts feature something that many junk foods do not -- great fat. Research indicates that polyunsaturated fat in walnuts may change the pathways for appetite and satiety.

And if you are concerned about calories, do not be! A 2012 research discovered a one-ounce serving of almonds (about 23 nuts) contains 20 percent fewer calories than recorded on the tag. Essentially, the chewing process doesn't fully split down the almond mobile walls, leaving some of the nut undamaged and unabsorbed through digestion.

10. Whole grains

Being on a diet and eating carbohydrates seem like they belong in 2 different buckets, but not necessarily! Whole grains are full of protein and fiber, so eating a bit goes a very long way in keeping you complete. Additionally, a fresh study indicates that eating whole grains rather than refined grains might rev your metabolism up. So, go on and consume your entire grains and venture from the comfort zone to try out farro, bulgur, spelled, Kamut, amaranth, millet, sorghum, or freekeh.

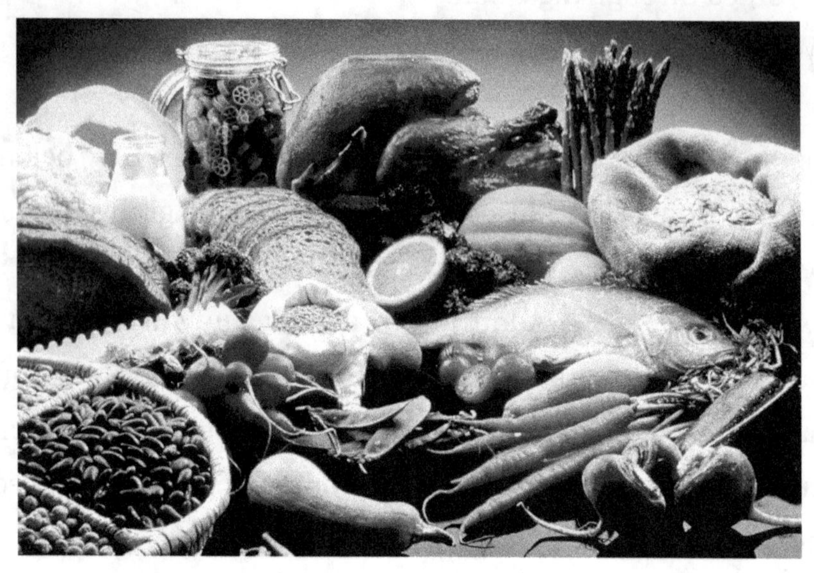

CHAPTER EIGHT
AUTOPHAGY AND INTERMITTENT FASTING

Nutrient deprivation is the essential activator of autophagy. Bear in mind that Glucagon is sort of the reverse hormone. It is like the game we played as children --'other day'. If insulin moves up, glucagon goes right down. If insulin goes, glucagon extends up. As we eat, insulin moves up and glucagon goes right down. As soon as we do not consume (quickly) insulin goes and glucagon goes upward. This increase in glucagon stimulates the process of autophagy. Fasting (increases glucagon) and supplies the best-known increase to autophagy.

Fasting is really a lot more beneficial than simply stimulating autophagy. It does two great things. By stimulating autophagy, we're clearing out most of our old, junky proteins and mobile components. At precisely the exact same period, fasting also stimulates growth hormone, which educates our body to begin generating some new snazzy elements for your system. We're giving our bodies the comprehensive renovation.

You want to eliminate the old things before it's possible to put in new things. Believe about renovating your kitchen. In case you've got older 1970s style lime green cupboards sitting about, then you must trash them prior to placing in some new ones. Hence that the practice of destruction (elimination) is equally as critical as the process of production. If you tried to install new cabinets without even taking out the previous ones, then it would not seem so sexy. So, fasting can in certain manners reverse the aging process, by eliminating older mobile crap and substituting it with fresh pieces.

An extremely controlled procedure

Autophagy is a highly controlled process. If it runs amok out of control, this could be harmful, therefore it must be carefully controlled. In mammalian cells, complete depletion of amino acids is a very powerful sign for autophagy; however, the use of individual amino acids is significantly more changeable. On the other hand, the plasma amino acid levels change only a bit. Amino acid signs and growth factor/insulin signs are believed to converge about the mTOR pathway -- sometimes known as the master regulator of nutrient signaling.

Thus, during autophagy, older mobile parts are broken down into amino acid parts (the building block of proteins). What happens to those amino acids? At the first stages of starvation, amino acid levels begin to rise. It's believed that those amino acids derived from autophagy are sent to the liver for gluconeogenesis. They may also be separated into sugar during the tricarboxylic acid (TCA) cycle. The next possible destiny of amino acids is to be integrated into new proteins.

The effects of amassing old junky proteins throughout the area can be viewed in two chief states -- Alzheimer's Disease (AD) and cancer. Alzheimer's Disease requires the accumulation of strange protein, either amyloid-beta or Tau protein that gums up the mind system. Though we do not yet have clinical trial proof for this, it might make sense that a procedure like autophagy that has the capability to clean out old protein can stop the progression of AD.

What ends autophagy? Eating, Insulin, or diminished glucagon. And proteins turn off this self-cleaning procedure. Plus, it does not take much. Even a little bit of amino acid (leucine) could stop autophagy chilly. This process of autophagy is exceptional to flaxseed -- something not seen in simple calorie restriction or dieting.

There's a balance. You get ill from a lot of autophagy, just as much as from too little. That gets us back into the organic cycle of existence -- feast and quick. Not continuous dieting. This allows for cell development during ingestion, and mobile cleansing through fasting -- equilibrium. Life is about balance.

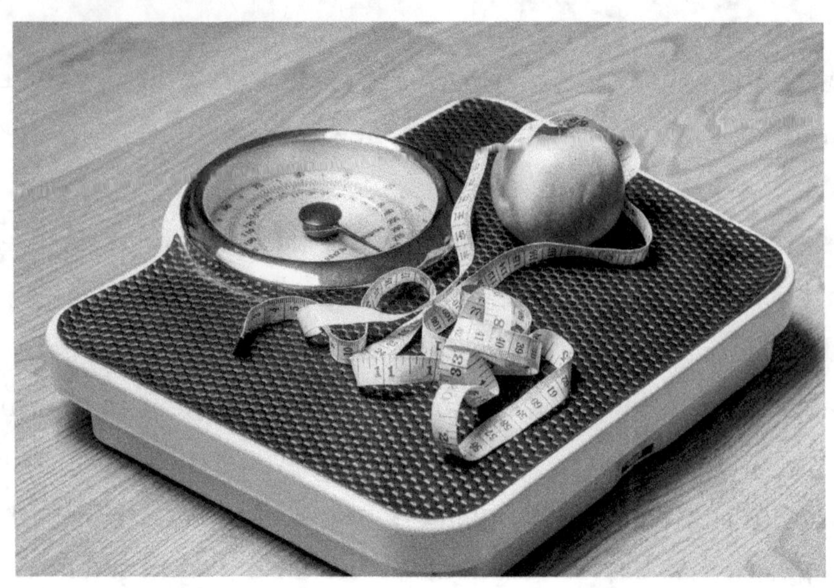

CHAPTER NINE
ANTI-AGING POWER OF AUTOPHAGY

Wellness -- we all desire this, and if you are a regular reader of the site, or simply wellness-curious, chances are, that you have got any sort of deal on the essentials such as fresh diet, fantastic sleep, motion, and normal comfort. This holistic approach is the road to feeling good and living well for as long as you can. However, there's another piece of this puzzle that is beginning to find some pleasant attention. That is autophagy. Auto-what? Researchers have known about it right from the'60s, but today it is starting to blossom in public awareness, partly as a result of recent discoveries about the mechanics for autophagy from Nobel Prize-winning scientist Yoshinori Ohsumi. But beyond the laboratory, what exactly does autophagy mean to you? For starters, better health; for others, a negative means of slowing down aging. Sound great? Then here is an introduction for this health wonder:

Autophagy -- it is your body's mobile recycling program. You might recall the word from high school chemistry? Ok, probably not. Well, autophagy is the own body's mobile house-cleaning system. It is a process that breaks down sub-part cells, so the banged-up ones who are not functioning well, then salvage the rest bits, recycling the elements to help construct new, new, healthy cells. This stripping of components and regenerating them moves on continuously inside your cells at varying rates. If your cells are receiving what they want in relation to the nutrients which fuel energy generation, autophagy hums along in reduced, maintenance level rate. But when things are not going so well and your cells are worried by nutrient deficiencies, viral germs, neglecting subcellular parts, etc., autophagy rises to the event and kicks into top gear. The uptick helps clear out the garbage -- i.e., the underperformers, the infected tissues, mobile toxins, etc. -- to help protect the rest of your healthy cells from damage, which then helps lengthen lifespan, slow the aging process and reduce disease threat.

Autophagy -- what is in it for you? A lot! Autophagy's got its hands in all, cellularly talking, providing an impressive collection of preventative and protective benefits from head to toe. One of the large bonuses, autophagy assists to
modulate inflammation, fostering it as needed to fight pathogens, and reducing it as needed, so cells do not stay in an infected condition forever; thus, suppressing chronic inflammation,

promote brain health and protect from Alzheimer's, Parkinson's and dementia, by removing the misshapen proteins whose accumulation is associated with the development of neurological ailments, combat infectious diseases, by eliminating illness-inducing microbes from within the tissues, clearing toxins, regulating inflammation and helping to keep immunity powerful,

stop metabolic breakdown, such as obesity and diabetes by boosting mobile health and turnover,

improve muscle operation, by substituting the cells which have been worn out or 'stressed' by exercise, using new, healthy cells.

When you put these advantages together, you are looking at possibly, among the most effective anti-aging packs anybody can ask for: a healthy mind, balanced metabolism, less chronic inflammation, stronger resistance, and much more resilient muscles.

Autophagy --provide you a kickstart. Granted, autophagy is happening all the time on your cells, however, there is a range of natural, wholesome ways that you may help ramp up the taking-out-the-garbage process. Listed below are a couple of ways you can help fire the autophagy incinerator:

Eat more autophagy-friendly spices -- Like curcumin, ginger, ginseng

Drink autophagy-boosting teas -- Like green tea and ginseng tea

Dig into autophagy-stimulating foods -- like coconut oil, broccoli, green peas, pomegranates.

Get into the routine, (although not surplus) intermittent fasting -- that, thanks in part to this dearth of incoming nourishment, worries the body and stimulates autophagy regardless of the temporary nutrient dip.

Attempt a ketogenic, or quite a low carb diet -- by supplementing carbohydrate ingestion; cells are made to utilize fat as their fuel, sending your body into ketosis, a change which can help boost autophagy, besides assisting body-fat reduction and lowering diabetes risk.

Insert some aerobic workout -- such as powerwalking, jogging, swimming laps; so, all this stress your body in a fantastic manner, and in so doing, ends up that autophagic warmth.

Do not forget to load up on good, quality sleep -- just in case you wanted yet another reason to get your match: autophagy also happens during sleep, so make your rest and allow your cells to clean out the cobwebs as you snooze.

Insert autophagy-supportive nutritional supplements -- such as omega-3 fish oils, vitamin D, MCT Oil

Run cold and hot -- like in alternating steam or sauna room time with cold showers; equally hot and cold pressure the cells, boosting autophagy.

While our scientific comprehension of autophagy continues to evolve, the main point is that autophagy-supporting behaviors -- such as a fantastic diet, sleep, motion, and nutritional supplement program -- are great, anti-aging, and health habits, which all of us should put to operate for the support for our bodies each day; right from now!

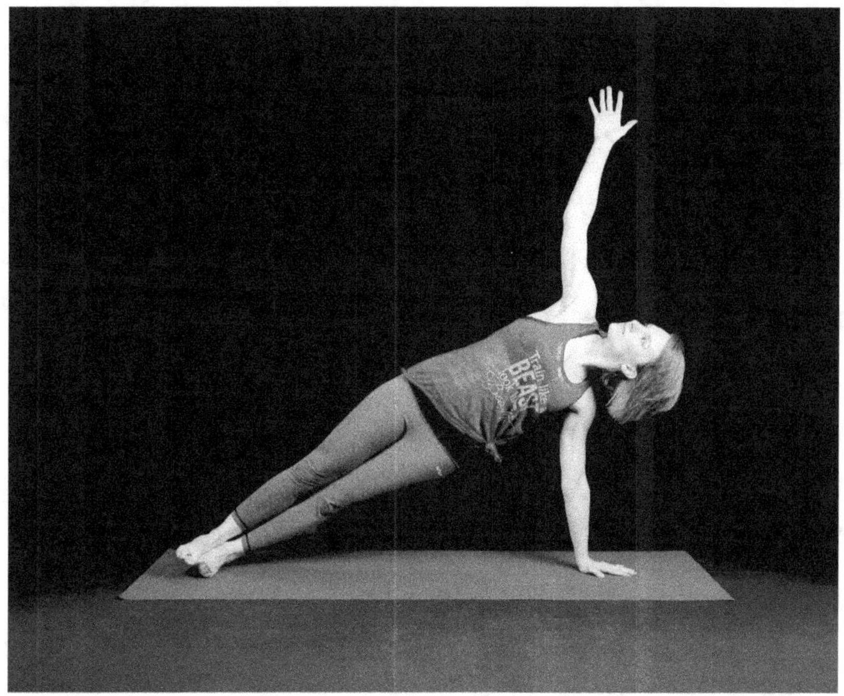

CHAPTER TEN
HOW TO INCORPORATE AUTOPHAGY IN DAILY LIFE

You will find many approaches in which you may turn your body's autophagy procedure (which doesn't have anything to do with juice cleanses). To cleanse your tissues and decrease inflammation, and keep your body functioning in tiptop shape, consider these five easy actions to grow the autophagy procedure. Remember that since autophagy is a response to anxiety, you must fool your body into believing it is a bit under siege. Here is the way:

1. Eat a high fat, low-carb diet

The change from burning glucose (carbohydrates) into ketones (fats) that happens to a keto diet mimics what happens naturally in a state -- and this raises autophagy.

2. Process a protein quick

One or two times every week, restrict your daily protein intake to 15-25 grams every day. This gives your body a complete day to recycle carbs, which will decrease inflammation and cleanse your tissues with no muscle loss. In this time period, whilst autophagy becomes activated, your body is made to absorb its own toxins and proteins.

3. Exercise Intermittent fasting

By skipping breakfast and eating all your meals in an abysmal window, you increase your own body's inherent autophagy procedure. Just like protein-specific quick, intermittent fasting provides your body an opportunity to "catch up" on those pesky toxins -- by cleaning up in real-time. Eliminate toxin build-up, by having a 16-28 hour quick.

If performed incorrectly, intermittent fasting may lead to hormone imbalances in girls. That is because girls are exceptionally sensitive to indications of starvation or calorie restriction. To sidestep problems, eat a fat-only breakfast, such as Bulletproof coffee. By removing carbohydrates and protein from your meal, you stay in a fasting condition, whereas the fat informs your body that you are not hungry. Read more about the way girls can exercise intermittent fasting.

4. Exercise utilizing high-intensity interval training

HIIT (high-intensity interval training) exercise is just another valuable approach to excite autophagy. Bear in mind that autophagy is a physiological reaction to anxiety, and high-intensity workout puts you at the good-stress sweet place since it worries you enough to excite the biochemical shift. You will become only enough impact loaded to make your muscles more powerful (and cause autophagy) without injury. Aim for about 20-30 minutes per day to allow your longevity an optimum increase.

5. Get Cosmetic sleep

When you know which sleep style you are, you can put yourself up to trigger autophagy throughout your circadian rhythms, or adrenal tissues.

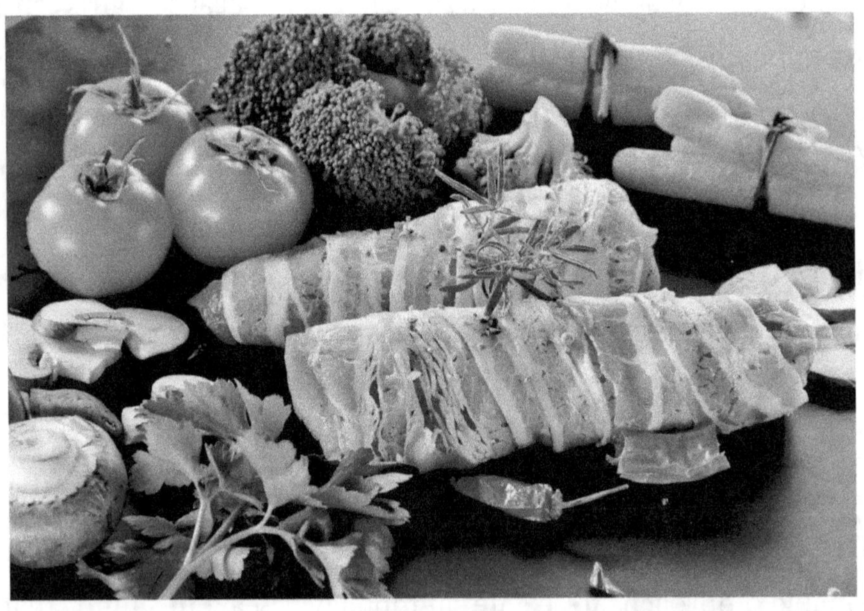